Praise for
Living in Limbo

"Michaels and Zilber, two consummate professionals, have constructed a work full of practical advice, common sense approaches, and loving spirit that will help anyone who is dealing with loss. I highly recommend this wise book—it will make your life easier and better."

—*Martin Blaser, MD, author of* Missing Microbes, *professor of medicine at NYU School of Medicine, and former chair of the Board of Scientific Counselors of the National Cancer Institute*

"This book is an invitation to a clarifying dialogue between two women who embrace life's ambiguity and urge readers to be honest when facing the challenges of unknowing. In the context of life threatening illness, they see life not death. Laura and Claire offer wisdom from their experience to grow responses that trust inner strengths and recruit external support."

—*David Cooper, former executive director of Colorado Regional AIDS Interfaith Network*

"Dealing with a loved one's serious illness can be one of the most unsettling situations we deal with in our lives, leaving us feeling lost and alone. This profound book steps in to provide clear, compassionate, and wise guidance for getting through the hard times. The book's innovative approach integrates both the expertise of a psychiatrist and the real life insights of someone who has been there. It provides practical advice for navigating the challenges of caregiving, as well as supportive, evidence-based counsel for coping emotionally and spiritually. If you are caring for a family member or close friend facing a health crisis, this is a book you will want to keep close at hand! You will open it again and again, relieved to have this "companion" assist you as you navigate through the limbo."

—*Susan Freeman, rabbi, professional chaplain, and pastoral educator*

D1550447

"The craftsmanship of *Living in Limbo* is the way that it creates a fugue between the voices of Michaels and Zilber, the antiphonal call-and-response between Michaels's remembrances as well as her subsequent insightful reflections upon those experiences, and Zilber's supporting analyses and interpretations which draw upon both science and spiritual wisdom. Part of the mastery of this book is that it mixes in equal doses the *expertise* that only can come from decades of clinical and psychotherapeutic experience, the *wisdom* that Michaels and Zilber have earned both professionally and in their personal lives with seriously ill loved ones, and the *love* that comes from deep care and openheartedness to the impermanence that *is* this precious life."

—*J. Jeffrey Franklin, PhD, associate vice chancellor at University of Colorado–Denver*

"When my husband was undergoing chemotherapy, I felt like I was supporting him by taking care of myself, our children, and the home and leaving him free to care for himself. Then I read *Living in Limbo* and realized how much I had let us both down. After a few tears, he and I were able to talk with open hearts about all of our feelings during that stage of his illness, for the first time. Then, when we found out that the illness had recurred and he would need a second round of treatment, and later a third, we were able to face our work together, in full partnership. The illness ended up strengthening our relationship, and we became better at loving each other and finding acceptance and even gratitude for the illness."

—*Judy Lucas, LMT in palliative care*

Living in Limbo

Living in Limbo

CREATING STRUCTURE AND PEACE
WHEN SOMEONE YOU LOVE IS ILL

Dear Carol,

May the lessons in this book be useful to you when you travel through limbo. —— Claire Zilber

Dear Carol -

Thank you for being part of my community during my time of limbo. —

With love,
Laura

Laura Michaels, MA, JD and Claire Zilber, MD

The identifying details in the vignettes and examples included in this book, other than Laura's personal story and journal entries, have been altered to protect the privacy of friends, acquaintances, colleagues, and patients.

ISBN: 1544242018
ISBN-13: 9781544242019
Library of Congress Control Number: 2017903779
CreateSpace Independent Publishing Platform
North Charleston, South Carolina

Contents

Introduction—Laura

This is not a club you wanted to join; none of us do. But in time, most of us will. Finding out that your loved one has a serious illness, injury, or disability changes you in a fundamental way. Your first reaction is probably "no": No, it can't be. No, that must be wrong. No, not him, not her. (No, not me.) You yearn for a cosmic remote control with which you can rewind to *before*, that time of relative, oblivious ease only revealed as such by the power of retrospect. In an instant, you feel transformed, alien to the identity and assumptions that shored you up only moments before.

When my husband, Bill, was diagnosed with lung cancer at the age of fifty-two, it felt as though life as we knew it came to a screeching halt. Everything we had always believed, all our assumptions, were instantly turned inside out and upside down. At the time, our children were fifteen, twelve, and six—smack in the middle of a contented childhood. Struggling with my shock and despair, I looked for books that would speak to me as I tried to make sense of and reorder my world.

So much has been written about illness from every conceivable angle, but in the overabundance of print and online resources, I didn't find what I needed—a guidebook for me, devastated by my husband's diagnosis. I was forced to move quickly into a cognitive and emotional place where I could cope most effectively with the minefield we had abruptly entered. Ultimately, I collected an assortment of tools from readings, wise people in my life, and inner strength I didn't even know I had. My goal in writing this book is to convey the techniques I collected and developed in this challenging time and make them readily accessible for others.

I feel both inspired and humbled by the thought that my experience might, in some small way, touch another person facing a similar challenge. I have spent most of my career in the field of mental health. My work has been primarily in advocacy and administration, but I am now engaged in a rewarding second career in mental-health counseling. While my career and education have given me insights into the issues we explore in this book, the examples I share are personal rather than professional; I am someone who has been "there," however you want to describe that particular place.

My conviction that an expert clinical perspective would be invaluable to this project led me to ask a psychiatrist friend and colleague, Claire Zilber, MD, for whom I have tremendous admiration and respect, to collaborate with me. In order to retain our own voices and perspectives, we have chosen to contribute complementary pieces with differentiated fonts representing each of our voices.

Who is this book for?

Simply put, if someone you love has been diagnosed with a serious illness, injury, or disability, this is for you. In cases where you are the parent, spouse, partner, child, brother, or sister of a person with an illness, it is quite likely that you will be involved, at some level, with the care of your relative. There are also situations when you may find yourself being that closest person, or one of the closest people, to a friend, coworker, grandparent, aunt, uncle, cousin, or neighbor. Not everyone has a family member or obvious choice for a caregiver who is willing and able to assume this role. Sometimes the person who seems most likely to take leadership and responsibility is physically, mentally, or emotionally incapable of doing so. With a myriad of family and community configurations in our society, the picture of who is in the front passenger seat with us on life's journey is not always evident or even static.

Although I offer many examples from my experience, the aim of this book is not to tell a story about my family and me. Not all the topics we explore will ring true for every reader; however, our goal is to present some of the universal themes and challenges that characterize the experience of caring for a loved one with an illness, injury, or disability. I am not asserting that there is only one right way (or wrong way) to react or respond, but in the places where I do strike a chord for you, perhaps these chapters will lend some structure to the turbulence you are confronting and will present some useful strategies and support as you travel this new frontier. Accept what works for you, and reject what doesn't, as you come to your own place and make decisions about how to approach this time in your life.

That said, while I know different people respond to crises in different ways, I wouldn't be writing a book if I didn't believe that certain attitudes and adaptive behaviors promote healthy coping, just as certain patterns and traps can make you more miserable. So when I fall into second-person commands, such as "Avoid" or "Don't," these are as much observations, even reminders, to myself as they are recommendations to anyone else. An example is my goal to be resilient; although this is a universal aspiration, it will look and feel different to each person who achieves it. In other words, we do have a destination of sorts in mind (i.e., peace, equanimity, joy), but there are as many ways to find it as there are people.

To express most authentically some of my thoughts and processing, I have included excerpts from my journal. Throughout Bill's illness, I often found a quiet sanctuary in the privacy of my little spiral notebook. It became a way for me to name, and even discover, some of the feelings I was experiencing. Although I hesitate to expose entries so personal and raw, there are emotions and perceptions that just do not translate with the same intensity and clarity when I paraphrase them now. Given that I explored certain ideas in my journal more than others, my quotes will appear where relevant and will address certain themes more than others. The "me" of today has a different perspective from the "me" at that time, and to whatever extent this difference in perspective might be useful to you, I have preserved that dynamic. These selections appear in italics.

Although the experience I describe in this book concerns my husband's battle with cancer, I have also dealt with grave and fatal illnesses affecting both my parents and other very close loved ones. Most of us will find ourselves in supporting roles multiple times throughout our lives, sometimes (as in my case) simultaneously or in quick succession, which compounds the need to garner coping skills strong enough to face the layers of these challenges.

The philosophical and practical approaches discussed here are meant to be applicable whether you are supporting someone facing brain injury, cancer, ALS, mental illness, Alzheimer's disease, HIV/AIDS, or any other acute or chronic illness or physical or mental disability. You may find this book helpful even if you are no longer caring for someone but have previously shared this experience. I believe that ultimately we all aspire to live with awareness and purpose, regardless of whether we are in crisis or in an uneventful, peaceful place.

The reality is that we all live, to some extent, in a state of impermanence; certainty of the future is beyond our control. Some of us are just more conscious of this truth because it has been shoved harshly in our faces. As I had various realizations throughout the process of my husband's illness, I wished I had had the benefit of some of these insights earlier in my life. Who among us wouldn't want to live more fully, more authentically, more in the present? So often we are waiting to reach a specific milestone until we can be happy or fulfilled. We fixate on a time in the future when things are going to be better: when I get a new job, when I find a partner, when the kids are grown, when I retire—when, when, when.

After diagnosis, you no longer have the luxury of postponing the task of evaluating the way you live your life on a daily basis. I am grateful that urgency helped me structure my thoughts and emotions so I could cope and thrive during the most challenging time of my life.

Introduction—Claire

It is my opinion that man is rather staggeringly endowed with adaptive capacities, and I am quite certain that when a person is clear on the situation in which he finds himself, he does one of three things: he decides it is too much for him and leaves it, he handles it satisfactorily, or he calls in adequate help to handle it. And that's all there is to it.
—Harry Stack Sullivan

have been interested in how people cope with and respond to illness since I was in medical school. I remember my very first clinical encounter as a second-year medical student, when I was assigned to interview a woman hospitalized with cancer. She was about the same age as my mother, whose sisters had both battled cancer successfully. I was intensely curious about whether this woman felt that her role as a mother to young adult daughters had been changed by her illness. Unfortunately, my questions were very upsetting to her, and I was banned from her room after the first interview. Thus I learned that my patients' interests must always come before my own and that I must follow their lead in deciding where to take the discussion.

Since that early lesson in tact, I have had the benefit of thousands of encounters with people who are coping with their own or a loved one's mental and medical illness. Early in my third year of medical school, I had a career-changing experience with a man with AIDS. From the first time

I met him until the end of his life, I saw how he was shunned by medical providers, hospital employees, and society in general. My curiosity about and sympathy for this man's experience allowed me to draw toward him at the same time that everyone else seemed repelled. This was a gift for us both. I was able to offer him some humanity and comfort, and he kindled my career interest in working with people with AIDS and other life-threatening or chronic illnesses.

After residency, I started a mental-health program for men and women with HIV infection, which I ran for eighteen years at the University of Colorado medical center. I also taught medical students, residents, nurses, pastoral counselors, and physicians, and I treated a wide range of patients. Now, in addition to my private practice, where I combine psychotherapy and pharmacotherapy to help my patients, I teach professional ethics for healthcare providers. I have been privileged to listen to people with acute and chronic medical illnesses, as well as people whose spouses, parents, or children were acutely or chronically ill, and I have learned a lot about the range of coping styles people employ when dealing with this unique kind of stress.

As editor of the Colorado Psychiatric Society's newsletter and chair of its ethics committee, I had the pleasure of working with Laura for twenty years in her capacity as the executive director of the society. Laura and I were colleagues and friends while she dealt with Bill's illness. She was always dignified yet never aloof. She responded with honesty to my questions, and she seemed to be in touch and at peace with her feelings.

Her demeanor seemed to stand in stark contrast to the angst I'd experienced when my own husband had been ill a decade earlier. At that time, I had struggled with self-pity and a lot of anxiety. I was stuck on the belief that what was happening to my young family was not fair until I finally realized fairness was an irrelevant concept. I wish I had had access to Laura's wisdom back then, so I am very pleased to be collaborating with her to bring inspiration and advice to other people walking a similar path.

My contributions to this book offer an objective counterpart to Laura's story and insights. My intention is to provide philosophical or clinical commentary for the personal experiences Laura describes. I include vignettes from my work with patients, although the identities of individuals and details of their experiences have been substantially altered to protect their privacy. I hope this book will help you find some new strategies for relaxing into your limbo experience so that you can move through it with more grace and find moments of stillness, peace, and joy.

Consider this book an open closet. Laura has filled the closet with clothes of many fabrics, styles, and colors, and I offer a set of hangers on which to arrange them. We invite you to try on our ideas for size. Keep those that suit you and leave the rest.

Note to Readers:

The authors' voices are distinguished in this book by layout and font. Sections written by Laura Michaels are in the standard body of the text, while Claire Zilber's contributions appear in the inset passages. The italicized pieces are reproduced from Laura's journal.

CHAPTER 1
Embracing Uncertainty

Unexpected illness brings with it a tsunami of uncertainties, from the nature of the problem, its treatment, and its prognosis to the ways in which one's life will need to be rearranged to adapt to temporary or permanent changes in the ill person's functioning. This can be incredibly stressful, but stress can serve as a catalyst for growth. Adaptation to stress, the basis for natural evolution, also can be a spark for personal transformation.

The Unknowable Future

> *Even cowards can endure hardship; only*
> *the brave can endure suspense.*
> —Mignon McLaughlin

Grammie used to talk about her life in chapters. She had her chapter where she was married and raising children. Then she had her husband's protracted illness and death. Then she had her career as an interior designer. And finally, she had her retirement and travels around the world. She viewed each chapter as unique, rich, and meaningful.

I have had my chapter of Bill and me in good health, raising our kids together while working and enjoying friends and family. Now I am in the chapter of dealing with his illness. My anxiety comes from two things: 1) I don't know how long this chapter will last or what its outcome will be and 2) I don't know what the next chapter will look like.

I keep wanting to jump ahead to the next chapter and see what is there. Is it back to Bill and me leading our lives with Bill in remission? Or is it me alone? The anxious part of me wants to peek at, anticipate, that chapter so that I can prepare for it. But the reality is that it hasn't been written yet. Even the chapter I'm in hasn't been written past the page I'm on. All I can do is keep going forward, page by page.

Life has a way of throwing us wild surprises. When Bill and I were struck completely unexpectedly with his diagnosis, it seemed inconceivable that we—*we*—could be in this position. We couldn't wrap our heads around this absurd news. It seemed absolutely illogical and unreasonable to us that our family was facing this particular crisis. Not that we felt superior or immune to the random instances of bad luck that befall some people, but this particular blow was stunning. Advanced lung cancer, out of the blue, three weeks after Bill had successfully completed his twenty-fifth marathon? With his robust lifestyle and upbeat spirit, Bill seemed to be the healthiest person around. A complete and devastating bombshell to our also youthful and energetic friends, it was a sobering concept. If Bill could become sick, anyone could.

Even before the initial shock had dissipated, we had to jump into action. Time was not on our side, and the situation demanded that every ounce of our energy be immediately transferred to dealing with Bill's cancer. We could not afford to allow our disbelief and grief to paralyze us.

Like most people, I have witnessed and experienced many situations in which I have been forced to integrate events that don't make sense to me. I have known young children who have died as the result of illnesses or accidents. I have known young adults who have had to cope with life-changing disabilities and unforeseeable tragedies. So why does it still always shake me to my core when life egregiously deviates from the path I expect? Why do most people appear to harbor expectations that life will take a predictable course when there is so much evidence to the contrary?

Some years ago, my father developed serious vascular disease. At one point, he suffered an aortic aneurysm most doctors would have considered irreparable. We were fortunate that a top vascular surgeon practiced in our area and was willing to attempt a cutting-edge but extremely difficult and risky procedure. This innovative operation was so successful that my father became the subject of a medical-journal article. In the ensuing years, he continued to have many health problems and was a frequent visitor to doctors and hospitals, but my father continued to surpass all predictions for his life expectancy.

Meanwhile, this prominent surgeon was at the pinnacle of his life and career, a pioneer in his field. He was vibrant and athletic, a strong contrast to most of his patients. One day we were shocked to read that this doctor had been killed in a diving accident. It was so improbable that my father, who had been critically ill more times than we could count, was plugging along, while the man who had literally saved his life was stricken in the prime of life. While we of course were grateful for my father's survival through so much medical adversity, this course of events was a stark example of how irrational and random life can be.

When life takes an unexpected turn, you may feel that your assumptions about the future were only illusory. On the other hand, you may end up having the future you anticipated all along. People do recover, go into remission, and surprise everyone. Your loved one might be in this category. I remember an old family friend who loved to tell the story about shopping for a life-insurance policy when he was a young man. At the time, he had several acquaintances in the insurance business, but none of them would sell him a policy, because he had a heart condition. At his seventy-eighth birthday party, he made what became a legendary quip in our family: "You know all those guys who wouldn't write me a life-insurance policy?" Pause. "They're all dead."

Living in Limbo

Life to me is defined by uncertainty. Uncertainty is the state in which we live, and there is no way to outfox it.
—Thomas H. Cook

I can't believe I'm having conversations using terms like "survival rates." It all feels so surreal, like my whole life is on hold. But this is my life, and there is no pause or rewind or fast-forward. It's all in play.

My grandmother died at eighty-nine while playing bridge. She was on vacation in North Carolina in seemingly remarkable health when she bid her three no-trump, won her hand, put her head down on the table, and that was that. Isn't this what we all secretly desire and even subconsciously expect? Living into old age with few health complaints, being active and productive, culminating in sudden and painless death? No heartbreaking diagnoses, CT scans, second opinions, hospital waiting rooms, oxygen, wheelchairs, nursing care, and terrifying limbo. No thought-controlling, appetite-erasing, panic-inducing, fear-breeding, all-encompassing, un-relenting limbo. Unfortunately for most of us, the circumstances of my grandmother's death are more the exception than the rule. More of us will deal with a difficult illness at some point.

I came up with the title of this book long before I ever wrote a sentence. To me, the concept of limbo accurately conveys the state of uncertainty I felt while I was coping with my husband's illness. To live in limbo is to dwell in a place that may feel transitional but in reality may range from days to decades.

Often when we think of limbo, we think of a status where things are put on hold *until* something else happens. We might say, "She was in limbo waiting for her visa to go through," meaning she couldn't work *until* an-other action occurred. Or, "He was in limbo waiting to hear about his financial-aid package," as in he couldn't choose his college *until* another decision was made. These contingent actions are not in our control. We are at the mercy of another occurrence paving the way for us to take our next step.

In dealing with Bill's cancer, I felt as though my life was or should be in suspension while the crisis played itself out. But I soon realized I couldn't stay on pause. I had to learn how to function even when I felt I was in psychological abeyance. I couldn't live my life waiting *until*. This position of uncertainty was a place where we were going to be parked for an indefinite period of time, so my mental effort had to focus on integrating this status into my reality. As contradictory as it sounds, I had to keep moving forward while stationed in limbo.

Most people who have been in a similar situation know the tension of waiting: waiting for a diagnosis, waiting for a test result, waiting for a treatment plan. And as is usually the case with a chronic or ongoing illness, just as one issue is resolved, you begin the wait for something else. The state of limbo usually has many layers. You may be in limbo awaiting a concrete item, such as what a biopsy will show. At the same time, you may feel you are in a vaster sense of limbo, wondering, *What is his/her/my/our future going to be?* Some of your questions will be answered in a matter of days; others may not be resolved in your lifetime. For me, the difficult task was learning how to manage this tension and incorporate it into the essence of my life.

I also found that in dealing with the course of an illness, life rarely follows a straight trajectory. You may think you have resolution, but then (for example) a week before a scheduled surgery, new information appears that makes the previous plan problematic. Countless variables must be assimilated and addressed. Tumors grow or shrink; experts disagree; side effects emerge.

The state of limbo you experience when your loved one is seriously ill can be completely disorienting. You don't know what the future will bring. Of course, you never did know that, but at some level you thought you did. You assumed that you would grow old with your spouse or partner, that your children would outlive you, that your parents would age well, and that siblings and close friends would be always by your side.

Living in limbo straps us on a roller coaster of emotions (concern, hope, frustration, fear, guilt) and often draws us into an exhausting vortex as we care for our loved ones. We may find ourselves racing from one specialist to another in a desperate search for the one answer that might change everything—or at least provide relief. The whirlwind experience of serious illness can take a catastrophic toll on both the patient and the caregivers.

> The word *limbo* was coined by Roman Catholic theologians in the Middle Ages to denote the border zone where innocent souls remain if they cannot enter heaven but do not deserve hell.[1] Limbo is an intermediate state. At times during the course of helping a loved one through a crisis, you may encounter limbo-like states. The period of waiting for a diagnosis or waiting to see if a treatment has been successful may mimic the border between heaven and hell. When you find yourself in this border zone, it may help to remember that, unlike the limbo of Catholic theology, you are not going to be here for the rest of eternity.

Life Is a Process

> *Life is not a particular place or a destination. Life is a path.*
> —THICH NHAT HANH

My assumptions about my future have all been tossed in the air—tossed in the air with no sense of how or where I'll land.

In the first months following Bill's diagnosis, in addition to being consumed by anxieties and fears, I thought a lot about my destination, my destiny. Where was this new twist in the road going to take me? Over time I began to see that my voyage would not culminate with a specific

---

1 *American Heritage Dictionary*, 4th ed. (Random House: New York, 1992), 491.

end point. My destiny would not be revealed at a defined moment in Bill's illness, better or worse. Life is a journey, and we will never reach the end while we are alive.

I think about how my view of the family car trip matured over the years. When I was young, our family took a trip we all later agreed had been an ill-conceived choice for our particular set of travelers: two parents, one grandmother, and three girls looking to be entertained. While the adults (three in the front) were admiring the beauty of the Canadian and Alaskan wilderness, my sisters and I could focus only on who was trespassing over whose exact third of the back seat. Our sole curiosity through miles and miles of breathtaking vistas was whether we were "there yet."

As a parent, my experience was completely different. I treasured our car rides as a family as we listened to books on tape, recalled infamous moments in our collective memories, detailed story lines of movies or television series, sang to the radio, stopped for meals in strange towns, pored over maps, and debated preferable routes. When I was truly being in the moment of the car ride itself, the *there* became incidental. The interactions we experienced as a family, away from the work and school frenzy and electronic interruptions, reinforced our connectedness, our bond. The process of listening to one another, laughing, and sharing transcended physical location. In many ways, the true purpose of our journey had very little to do with reaching the final town on our itinerary.

> It is not what you attain but how you go about getting there that gives life meaning. Consider the process of therapy: Many people are under the mistaken impression that the healing comes from some weighty, wise words delivered by the therapist. In reality, the healing comes from the process of dialogue and interaction between patient and therapist.
>
> The act of describing your pain or fear or anger and of being listened to and understood helps to change the pain or fear or anger. Certainly the therapist may say something interesting or helpful or even profound, but the benefit is not from the words alone. The

experience of sharing your story with someone who is interested and who listens with empathy is deeper and more transformative than mere words. Together, patient and therapist bear witness to the suffering and thus overcome it.

So it is with life. Religions and philosophers have offered an abundance of guidelines for how to live—from how to treat our neighbors to what to do with our fear of the unknown and everything in between. It seems that no one is able to adhere to these sage tenets all the time, which is why we have rituals such as New Year's resolutions and Gutor (a Tibetan Buddhist holiday that occurs right before their new year), in which people deal with unfinished business and unhappy memories so they can approach the new year with gratitude, openness, and appreciation for the moment. Lent and Yom Kippur are scheduled opportunities to reflect on our shortcomings and rededicate ourselves to trying harder next time.

Through this annual self-evaluation and repair, we become slightly wiser, a little more prepared for life's challenges. Informally, this same process occurs in everyday life, in private thoughts and conversations with friends, after difficult interactions with family or co-workers, or whenever we feel inadequately prepared to respond gracefully to whatever is before us. With time and effort, our adjustments and adaptations help us mature into more effective, capable, resilient beings.

Life is a process of accumulated experiences from which we grow and evolve, and hopefully, we become more adept at navigating our way through the world. Illness, in oneself or a loved one, inevitably prompts reflection and growth. If we are lucky, we first meet serious illness remotely, perhaps in childhood through a distant relative or the relative of a friend. Gradually, as the young person travels along the path of life, he or she gets more glimpses of illness. If there is an opportunity to talk about these glimpses, to examine the feelings associated with loss and to assimilate them into the individual's understanding of the world, then the person will be better prepared to cope with the eventual serious illness of someone close, such as a parent, sibling, or life partner.

Sometimes a young person's first encounter with serious illness or death is too close or traumatic, such as losing a parent when the child is very young or witnessing a violent injury. The young psyche is not yet prepared for such an existential challenge. When that person meets illness in the future, the early traumatic feelings may reemerge and interfere with the ability to respond to the present situation. Psychotherapy can be very helpful in the processing of unresolved trauma and grief so that the individual is better able to encounter subsequent loss with more equanimity.

Security and Change

> *Security is mostly a superstition. It*
> *does not exist in nature.*
> —HELEN KELLER

Somehow I need to find stability in my instability, make my psychological limbo into a solid structure.

At our first meeting with the oncologist, Bill asked the doctor, "Am I going to die?"

"Yes," he replied. "And so will your wife, and so will I."

Although unexpected things had happened in my life, it wasn't until Bill's diagnosis that I had to painstakingly learn how to not know. It is difficult to fully accept the idea that we just can't have all the answers. Most of the answers we think we have, the assumptions we make, and our expectations for the future are fluid and unreliable, as ultimately they may or may not occur. But even with an awareness of this truth, I still find that the realization that I'm not in control never quite sinks in, despite constant reminders that I actually lack omnipotence. I seem to have an insatiable desire for a sense of security, even though I know this state of being is ephemeral and notoriously false.

The journey of life requires that we dwell in uncertainty, as uncomfortable as that may be. The state of not knowing may make us feel vulnerable and somehow in danger. When our sense of self becomes threatened by the fear we encounter, we may experience an emotional fight, flight, or freeze—and our instinct to protect ourselves sets in. We often end up assuming the worst to somehow immunize ourselves from the hurt we may encounter if our projections turn out to be true.

I remember once saying to a friend, "I just always want to know what is going to happen."

"Why?" she asked.

I waited a moment and was amazed to see that she was perfectly sincere in her question. *Why do I have this need to know?* I wondered. My friend claimed not to have this yearning, a declaration I found incomprehensible. It seemed unnatural to me that a person could lack a burning curiosity about what is next, but I envied her acceptance of this reality. The rational side of me was aware that we cannot know what is going to happen tomorrow, next week, or next year. And spending time anticipating, predicting, and longing to know what the future would bring was only wasting my precious energy and focus that belonged to the present.

After September 11, 2001, everyone in the nation was forced to confront the precariousness of life. Thousands of regular people doing regular things didn't come home that day, which had started out so ordinarily. We are living in a time when events with mass casualties are a reality, whether they are acts of violence or natural disasters, making naïve any complacent presumptions about our personal and national invulnerability. Our anticipated destinies are only that: anticipations. There are no guarantees. Even tragic, painful events must find their place in our lives.

And yet. Whenever I am inclined to live my life waiting for the proverbial ax to fall, I remind myself how paralyzing and fruitless that attitude is. Knowing that security is an illusion does not require that we live in fear of all the misfortunes or tragedies that possibly could befall us. It is a simple fact that we cannot know the course our lives will take, and because we cannot weave our own futures, we are forced to integrate unpredictability and insecurity as part of our life's fabric. We travel in a state of continuous change. That impermanence is what gives beauty and urgency to the present.

Change is perpetual. Heraclitus (535–447 BC) wrote, "Change alone is unchanging."[2] Ovid (43 BC–17 AD) agreed, "Nothing in all the world is free from change. All is a flux of forms that come and go."[3] To the extent that we are able to accept the impermanence inherent in life, we are better able to adapt to the inevitable flow of change.

In a world of constant change, uncertainty is inevitable. Erich Fromm, a noted twentieth-century psychologist, welcomed uncertainty as necessary for self-discovery and actualization. He wrote, "The quest for certainty blocks the search for meaning. Uncertainty is the very condition to impel man to unfold his powers."[4] Uncertainty and change are not only inevitable; they are useful. The Sanskrit mantra "Om nama shivaya" loosely translates to "Salutations to that which I am capable of becoming."[5] It is an expression of acceptance for one's personal, ongoing evolution.

Sometimes change is almost imperceptible. At first glance, a shoreline looks like it has been there forever, an eternal boundary

---

2 Heraclitus, quoted in Douglas Soccio, *Archetypes of Wisdom*, 9th ed. (Boston: Cengage Learning, 2016), 65.

3 Brooks Otis, *Ovid as an Epic Poet*, 2nd ed. (London: Cambridge University Press, 1970), p.82.

4 Erich Fromm, *Man for Himself: An Inquiry into the Psychology of Ethics* (New York: Routledge Classics, 2003), 32.

5 Thomas Ashley-Farrand, quoted by William Ferro, http://www.yogaflavoredlife.com/mantra-of-extraordinary-power/

between land and sea. The waves move in and out, and the birds circle overhead, but the beach appears constant. Yet we all know the sand is moving—eroding here, building up a sandbar there—in a subtle and continuous pattern of change.

So it is with our relationships. When we are in love, we want our relationship to stay just how it is forever. That would be impossible, even undesirable. New lovers are so absorbed with each other that they rarely have energy for other relationships. How could they take care of babies, raise children, or attend to careers if they remained focused only on each other? The relationship *must* change if it is to last and if the individuals in the couple are going to be able to continue to develop as adults. Couples who can adapt to change, who allow for each person's maturation, and who accommodate external changes—such as new jobs, shifting financial security, growing children, and aging parents—are more likely to experience enduring love than couples who cling tenaciously to their early romantic view of each other.

If the couple stays together long enough, inevitably one or both individuals will develop a life-threatening health problem. The couple's ability to adapt to this new challenge is likely to echo their response to previous challenges. If the husband felt abandoned after the baby was born, when the wife's attention had to be directed elsewhere, he may feel abandoned again when his wife turns her attention to her health problems. If the wife felt resentful that the husband's career absorbed the lion's share of his energy, she may feel angry or resentful now that his energy is diverted to doctor's appointments or lifestyle changes. If a person was often fearful that his or her partner would leave, the partner's illness is likely to rekindle and amplify that fear.

Does this mean that couples or parent-child dyads or siblings are doomed to repeat the same patterns of responses their whole lives? Thankfully, no. Everything always changes, and we can change, too. If we are uncomfortable with our feelings of abandonment, resentment, or fear, we can work to understand and change them. Sometimes this can happen simply through self-examination or talking to a partner or friend. Sometimes people find a therapist or clergy member to help them cope with and alter maladaptive responses. This is the beauty of getting older: we can learn to re-spond differently. We do not have to repeat the same old patterns of interaction that didn't go well the first time. Growth is hard, but it is good. Change is hard but also can be good. Om nama shivaya.

CHAPTER 2

Grounding Yourself

The shoe that fits one person pinches another;
there is no recipe for living that suits all cases.
—CARL JUNG

Some people might ask, if the future is unpredictable and change is inevitable, why bother trying at all? It is important not to misinterpret our inability to predict and control all outcomes as utter powerlessness. In reality, we have many choices about how to approach the challenges before us. In this chapter, we discuss these choices, such as adopting a mental attitude of hopefulness and paying attention to the language we use as we define problems. We can control how we think and talk about the illness and how we respond to other people's reactions.

Coping Styles

I want my lipstick to tell everyone in this room that I think
I have a future and I know I will wear lipstick again.
—GERALYN LUCAS[6]

No one can presume how another person might handle news of a difficult diagnosis. We are all individuals, and what works for me may feel

---

6 Geralyn Lucas, *Why I Wore Lipstick to My Mastectomy* (New York: St. Martin's Griffin, 2005).

inauthentic or counterproductive to you. Some people feel overwhelmed by their misfortune and want others to likewise view their circumstances as an unfair or tragic turn of events. Others adopt a hopeful, optimistic attitude and expect others to do the same. People often change their outlook from one direction to the other or to some place in between as they move through the journey. There is no right way.

As I consider my own situation and those of others I have known, I have noticed how coping styles may differ according to our underlying personalities or temperaments, the severity of the illness, and the degree of burden we are handling physically or emotionally. Some of us have previously dealt with challenging limbo circumstances. For others, this is the first time we are being tested to such a degree. Sometimes we rise to the occasion. Sometimes we fall apart. Some of us cope by not thinking about the situation and trying to deflect conversation and attention away from the illness. Others of us process nonstop, our minds involuntarily perseverating. In my experience, I found myself moving in and out of each of these categories, as internal and external variables were ever fluid.

Illness is a moving target. Just when you think you have a handle on things, they may change, perhaps causing a corresponding shift in your attitude or ability to cope. Such variables may include the duration of the illness; the way it affects regular life activities; the degree of pain or discomfort of your loved one; and your loved one's attitude, ability to handle treatment, and interactions with others.

> It may be challenging for those who are caring for a medically or psychologically ill person to move along their own paths in sync with the pace of the person who is ill. Certainly it would be remarkable if everyone in the family and circle of friends were all at the same point on each of their personal paths, each able to understand and accept the choices being made by the ill person right as they happen. It is more likely that people will walk their own paths at their own pace—some at a steady rate, others with stops and starts along the way. The differences in pacing may create conflict,

but if we acknowledge that these are merely variations in speed of adaptation and if we can be patient with the process, the conflict need not be severe.

In one family, the matriarch was slowly succumbing to vascular dementia. At first, the woman's grown children seemed more aware of her cognitive decline than did her husband, who protected himself and his wife by filling in her lapses during conversation. It was initially hard for him to accept the changes in his wife. During the long, middle part of her illness—after he had accepted the diagnosis but before death was imminent—the woman's husband paid careful attention to her needs. He developed systems for his caretaking so that his wife could expect things to happen in a predictable pattern.

As her abilities declined, the old systems wouldn't work as well, and he had to develop new ones. These were times of being temporarily out of sync until he could catch up to her on the path of her illness. Toward the very end of the woman's life, her husband, who had been the primary person taking care of her, was the first to recognize and accept that his wife's death was imminent. The children now lagged behind a bit, still urging their father to try a new medication, which he saw as irrelevant at this stage. Fortunately, this family had the ability to tolerate one another's different paces of acceptance, so the predominant feeling was one of support.

Most of the time, we will respond in a way that is consistent with who we have always been. But sometimes we may surprise everyone, including ourselves. A sunny personality may become bitter. A negative person may project uncharacteristic hope to his family. A lifelong competent person may become emotionally incapacitated and unable to function. All bets are off in this new frontier, but it is my experience and observation that we react in the way we usually tend to react.

In our case, Bill and I wanted to hear every success story, regardless of how random or far removed. As long as it included the phrases "lung cancer" and "still alive," we would hang on every word of the account. Someone would say, "My friend's father had lung cancer and was given six months to live; that was twenty-seven years ago, and he's still playing golf." We would repeat the story later to anyone who would listen. At the same time, my sister had a friend whose husband was going through cancer treatment, and he had no interest or patience with other people's stories. "That is irrelevant to my situation," he would say. "It means nothing to me." People are different, and there is no merit in trying to judge another's approach to a difficult life challenge.

When my younger daughter was in preschool, I met a mother whose son was severely disabled. He did not appear to have any voluntary movement or to be able to make a cognitive connection with others. I thought about how heartbreaking it would be to have a child who couldn't even make eye contact, let alone have a relationship with another person. But somehow this mother was cheerful as she took her son out into the world, a world of which he seemed to have no awareness. As she pushed him in his wheelchair, his head bowed, to various activities, she chose not to let these circumstances prevent her from participating fully in life.

Some people cope by being hyperfocused on the problem at hand, creating lists and charts to organize their thoughts and quell their anxiety. They may put the rest of their lives on hold. Others cope by focusing on the mechanics of day-to-day life, attending to their job and household responsibilities and not really thinking much about the crisis itself. Sometimes a couple will adopt opposite coping styles, which may create some conflict but be adaptive in the long run.

For example, when a young girl was diagnosed with a rare childhood cancer, her mother became very focused on work, because she knew that without the health insurance she had through her job, the family would not be able to afford the treatment and services her daughter required. She became more attentive to finances, insurance benefits, and other details than was her usual style. Her husband became almost exclusively focused on ushering his daughter through the health-care system. He quit his job and dedicated himself to caring for his child during the year of treatment she required.

Neither parent's coping style was a problem; in fact, they were both necessary and adaptive. Nevertheless, occasionally each adult would feel upset with the other, because previously their marriage had been fairly egalitarian regarding how they divided responsibilities, and now they were pushed into more extreme, nontraditional roles. Sometimes the mother felt guilty that she could not go to more medical appointments. Sometimes the father wished he could escape to an office. It helped them to recognize that both responses were necessary and that they had each gravitated to their respective coping strategies, based on long-standing personality strengths.

A very close friend told me that in a difficult time in her life, she imagined herself on a boat in a turbulent sea. Every now and then, she would find an island of tranquility, where she could feel normal, at peace, and even joyous. She encouraged me to try to find those islands in my life. I considered this but realized it worked better for me to reverse the visualization.

I decided to picture myself on a tranquil sea where I would encounter some islands of turbulence along the way. Maybe it wasn't a huge difference, but I needed the image that despite Bill's illness, the predominant part of my life was still positive. It depressed me to think of my life as perpetually cloudy with an occasional burst of sunshine. Had I carried the self-image of a weary sailor constantly battling hardships on the harsh sea, I think I would have become overwhelmed by the brutal conditions. By adjusting the mental image, I could put the challenges in the context of the rest of my life.

There are many personality domains that help determine our responses. One way of categorizing personality is the description of four temperaments. Alternatively, personality may be defined on the continuum of extroversion and introversion.

The Four Temperaments and their Coping Styles

Temperament theory was developed by the Greek physician Hippocrates (460–370 BC). He believed that certain human moods, emotions, and behaviors were caused by body fluids, or humors: blood, yellow bile, black bile, and phlegm. Galen (131–200 AD) further developed the temperament categories, which he labeled sanguine, melancholic, choleric, and phlegmatic. Avicenna (980–1037 AD) extended the theory of temperaments to include qualities of emotion, intellect, moral attitudes, self-awareness, and bodily movement.

Choleric

Originally used to describe a bitter-tempered person (in French, colère means anger), temperament theory recognizes the adaptive side of the choleric person's considerable energy. A person who is choleric has a lot of passion and ambition, which may explain why many charismatic military and political leaders share this temperament. A choleric person likes to be in charge and can dominate people of other temperaments, especially phlegmatic types, unless they learn to moderate their intensity. A choleric person copes with a problem by attacking it head-on. In a medical crisis, this person wants to know the exact treatment plan and will have a take-charge approach to care.

Melancholic

Melancholy is sadness or depression, but a person with a melancholic temperament is not necessarily sad or depressed.

Rather, a person with a melancholic temperament is often sensitive, thoughtful, and considerate of others. Melancholics can be highly creative in artistic forms of expression as a way of coping with tragedy and cruelty in the world. A melancholic person may also be a perfectionist. While this may lead to a strong sense of organization and self-sufficiency, a melancholic person may inadvertently shut out others while single-mindedly pursuing a goal. A person with a melancholic temperament may cope with a medical problem by attending to the scientific details of the pros and cons of treatment options, which can lead to being a well-informed patient.

Sanguine

The sanguine temperament is cheerful, emotionally expressive, outspoken, curious, and imaginative. People of a sanguine temperament tend to enjoy social gatherings and make new friends easily. They are usually quite creative and prone to daydreaming. Sanguine temperaments can also be very sensitive, compassionate, and thoughtful. Sanguine personalities generally struggle with following tasks all the way through, may be chronically late, and tend to be forgetful. In a medical crisis, people with a sanguine temperament may cope best by relying on their optimism about treatment and their friendly relationships with health-care providers, rather than focusing on the scientific details.

Phlegmatic

A person with a phlegmatic temperament tends to be calm, kindhearted, and content. They can be very accepting and affectionate. They may be shy and may prefer stability to uncertainty and change. They are relaxed, rational, curious, and observant; however, their resistance to change may lead them to have avoidant responses to conflict. A person with a phlegmatic temperament may cope with a medical crisis by being very compliant with treatment recommendations but may need encouragement to speak up when meeting with health-care providers.

While some individuals fit neatly into a single temperamental style, others are blends of two or more temperaments. It is useful to identify your temperament, because this can help you understand your strengths and weaknesses, your motivations and challenges. Similarly, understanding the temperament of people you love may help you appreciate their strengths, accept their weaknesses, and understand how to work most effectively with them in a medical crisis.[7]

Introversion and Extroversion

Introversion and extroversion are personality traits originally described by Carl Jung, a Swiss psychiatrist.[8] An extrovert tends to be outgoing and gregarious and feels energized by interacting with others. An introvert prefers time spent alone and is energized by thinking, reading, writing, or creating. Introverts are not necessarily shy or socially inept, but they are more likely to feel overwhelmed or depleted in large social gatherings, whereas extroverts tend to feel bored with too much time alone.

Most people have a blend of introversion and extroversion. Despite the linear appearance of the diagram that follows, introversion and extroversion probably do not exist on a continuum. Rather, Jung believed these qualities exist as two separate dimensions, with each person falling along a dimension of more-to-less extroversion and a separate dimension of more-to-less introversion and with one dimension more developed than the other.

For example, politicians or rock stars may be very well-developed in their extroverted qualities, which help make them dynamic and vibrant on stage in front of a crowd, but they may also have introverted qualities, such as the capacity for quiet thought when

---

7   Rudolf Steiner, *The Four Temperaments* (Forest Row, England: Rudolf Steiner Press, 2008).

8   Carl Jung, edited and translated by Gerhard Adler and R.F.C. Hull, *Psychological Types* (Princeton, NJ: Princeton University Press, 1971).

they seek inspiration for a speech or song. Conversely, a poet or a research scientist may have highly developed introversion traits, which make hours with pen and paper or in the laboratory pleasurable and productive. Simultaneously, they may have an extroverted side, competing in poetry slams or whooping it up at a ball game on weekends.

Extroverts, who thrive on interaction with others, are likely to want to share their crisis with a wide circle of friends and family in order to get as much support as possible. Introverts, who recharge their batteries through solitude and quiet, may conserve their energy by confiding in only a very few people. The approach you take should be determined by what feels comfortable and helpful to you.

When the person who is ill has a different coping style from the primary caretaker, it is often possible to find a compromise that works for both people. For example, if the person with the health crisis is an introverted and very private person and the partner is a social person with many close friends, they might agree on two or three people to whom the partner has permission to speak freely in exchange for reticence with everyone else. This solution respects both the patient's wish for privacy and the partner's desire for support.

People with sanguine or choleric temperaments tend to be more extroverted, while those with melancholic or phlegmatic temperaments may be more introverted. Jung also conceptualized a continuum of cognitive style, with some people processing information and making decisions primarily based on thinking and others more inclined to process based on feeling.[9]

---

9 Ibid.

Temperaments According to Their Cognitive Style and Degree of Introversion/Extroversion[10]

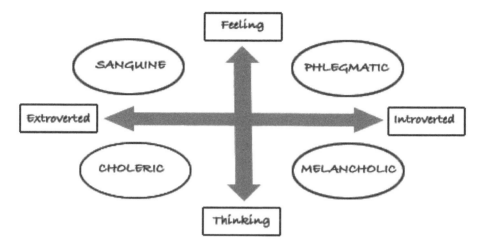

Sometimes the patient and the primary caregiver may have radically different preferences about how they want to think about and talk about what is happening. For example, a young woman with a sanguine temperament who had advanced multiple sclerosis (MS) was terrified of death and did not want to hear or talk about anything related to her dying. Her husband, who had a melancholic temperament, desperately wanted to talk to her about what was happening, but every time he tried to broach the subject, his wife became inconsolably anxious and upset.

She was soothed only by optimism, promises of new experimental treatments, rays of hope. He was too pragmatic to give her this reassurance; it felt like a lie to him. What she needed was someone who could project optimism. What he needed was someone who could tolerate hearing about his sorrow. Rather than getting one of them to change his or her approach, they each needed to find another person (a friend, family member, or therapist) who could honor their preferences and meet their respective needs for optimism or pragmatism.

---

10 Diagram created by John Menninger, 2015.

Making a Choice

> *Our unique opportunity lies in the way*
> *in which we bear our burden.*
> —VICTOR FRANKL

In his classic book *Man's Search for Meaning*, Victor Frankl recounts his time in a concentration camp in Nazi Germany. In order to cope with the horrors of his everyday life, he developed a philosophy based on his experience: Even when you are suffering, you still have a choice in how you approach the hardships you are enduring. Life continues to have meaning as you retain your faith in the future. He writes:

> We who lived in concentration camps can remember the men who walked through the huts comforting others, giving away their last piece of bread. They may have been few in number, but they offer sufficient proof that *everything can be taken from a man but one thing: the last of the human freedoms—to choose one's attitude in any given set of circumstances, to choose one's own way* (emphasis added).[11]

We all know we have little control over most of the things that occur in our lives. As Frankl so wisely observes, all we can truly control is the way we approach what is happening to us. We can choose how we respond to the events in our lives. None of us knows what the future will bring.

The ability to make choices is a power we crave from an early age. I remember as a parent of toddlers how it was necessary to give my children the sense that they could affect certain aspects of their lives. Maybe I wouldn't give them the choice of having soda or milk for dinner, but they could choose if they had their milk in the blue cup or the red cup. Even as adults, when our lives feel out of control, there are certain times when we can make clear choices, especially when it comes to the attitudes we assume and the perspectives we take. We can figure

---

11 Viktor E. Frankl, *Man's Search for Meaning* (Boston: Beacon, 2006), 65–66.

out which pieces of our lives are within our control and make an impact accordingly.

Not only can it be helpful to be deliberate in choosing how you respond to the news and implications of your loved one's illness, but you may also want to assert yourself early on through the tone you set with others. Bill decided from the beginning that he did not want to be inundated with an outpouring of sympathy. He sent a blast e-mail to everyone he knew, informing friends and acquaintances of his diagnosis and explaining that he was choosing to approach the situation in a positive way with hope and the intention to live his life to its fullest potential.

People responded accordingly and made a huge effort to allow their respect and deference to his simple request to outweigh their own fears and anxiety about the bad news. I imagine that in their own homes and to one another, friends expressed their skepticism about Bill's optimism. But in their interactions with us, for the most part, our family and friends complied with his wishes, even if that attitude may have felt contrived to them. The positive energy sent our way was of great comfort to both of us.

Managing Gracefully

> *You play the hand you're dealt. I*
> *think the game's worthwhile.*
> —CHRISTOPHER REEVE

I want to do so much more than cope with this situation. I want to cope well. I want to model coping for my children. I want to grow and surprise myself. To acknowledge my broken heart but not stay broken.

In *It's Easier Than You Think: The Buddhist Way to Happiness*, Sylvia Boorstein discusses the concept of "managing gracefully."[12] Many of us have burdens

---

12 Sylvia Boorstein, *It's Easier Than You Think: The Buddhist Way to Happiness* (San Francisco: Harper San Francisco, 1995).

and challenges in our lives, but in spite of these difficulties, we can be all right, especially when we learn to manage our stresses. Even if we don't feel great, we can still feel like we are managing. And managing gracefully is all the better.

When I first got a laptop, I briefly became a devotee of computerized card games. Fortunately it was an addiction I could easily conquer by deleting them entirely from the machine. But during that period of enchantment, I would eagerly log on to receive an electronically dealt hand to start off a new session of Freecell or Hearts. If I started out with cards I didn't like, I often immediately clicked to deal again so that my odds of winning were better (and presumably the game would be more fun). Sometimes I played the hand anyway and found that I actually received more gratification if I could win with what I believed to be a bad hand. As the well-established card-playing analogy goes, in real life, we can't simply choose to deal again; we have to play the hand we are given to the best of our ability, even if it is "bad."

As I attempted to approach our new life circumstances in a calm way, I had no better teacher than Bill himself. His innate optimism and self-contained equanimity were a huge contrast to my inner chaos. The fact that *he* was able to manage so effortlessly inspired me to follow his lead, however inept and unnatural I often felt. His positive attitude and philosophic composure kept his friends engaged and devoted, which fueled his energy and spirits. His warmth and their warmth fed each other in a circular harmony. To the extent that it is possible, managing gracefully is to everyone's benefit, including your own. It keeps you in karmic peace and prevents you from becoming isolated.

Of course, not every patient reacts the way Bill did, and there are clearly occasions when being warm and inviting is not possible or even desirable. There may be situations when you need to be demanding or protective or withdrawn. There may be times when you must fall utterly, completely apart into a thousand pieces. And there may be people who must be held at a safe distance. So I am *not* suggesting that you need to be a graceful, congenial host who eagerly welcomes people to your family's crisis. I *am* suggesting, though, that if you can get to a place where you are able to internalize the belief that you are going to be OK, it can give you strength as you move forward. And if you can impart that feeling in your interactions with other people, it can be beneficial to your social and emotional well-being.

I found this to be particularly important in my role as a parent. By modeling the attitude that *we* could handle this, I believe Bill and I greatly influenced our children's attitude that *they* could handle this. We continued to interact with each other as we always had, moving together in a positive direction toward the unknown future. The strength we derived from each other fed our inner strength and vice versa. A common metaphor for a family is that it is like a mobile hanging over a baby's crib. Each member is part of a system that is interconnected: when one dangling part is moved, the rest move, too. Notice these connections and interactions. It can be helpful to be aware of our own reactions when we are moved, as well as to be mindful of how our movements affect others.

Keeping Hope Alive

> *Hope means different things to different people, and different things to the same person as he/she moves through stages of illness. When we talk to patients and find out what is really worrying them, we can almost always give them realistic assurances.*
> —HOWARD BRODY

We try to stay encouraged that Bill will be one of those great success stories that have inspired us so much over the past few months. By now I have heard about more than a dozen people who were at stage IV, at a place where doctors barely had anything to offer, and now they're 3, 7, 15 years out and doing great. These are the stories that keep us going.

From the beginning, it was important for us to maintain hope. Even when the odds are terrible, *someone* has to be on the far right-hand side of the bell curve.

Hope can change over time. At first we may hope that there has been a mistake, that the diagnosis is wrong. This hope usually doesn't last too long as second opinions are offered and additional tests are completed. If you're reading this book, you likely have already seen this early hope extinguished. Next, we may move into hoping for a cure. We hope the illness or disability will be successfully treated to the point of disappearing or going into remission.

Often a cure isn't an option, so we hope treatment will make the condition better—or at least keep it stable. We hope it doesn't get worse. If it does, we may hope our loved one doesn't suffer. We hope symptoms can be comfortably managed.

Sometimes all we can do is hope for a miracle.

With all the dramatic progress being made in the field of medicine, I often wondered, how much can doctors know long range about someone at the time he or she is diagnosed? There are no data on someone who is diagnosed today. When his first treatment failed, Bill was able to get a new drug that hadn't even been available when he had received his diagnosis *six weeks* earlier. It is an exciting time for medical research and treatment, and each person and each situation is unique.

> One of the most basic concepts in science and statistics is the bell-shaped curve. Many measurable phenomena, if plotted on a graph, fall into a bell-shaped curve, with most of the observations in the middle, tapering off at both ends. For example, if we measure the height of twenty-five-year-old, white, American men and graph the results with number of men on the vertical axis and number of inches on the horizontal axis, it might look something like this:

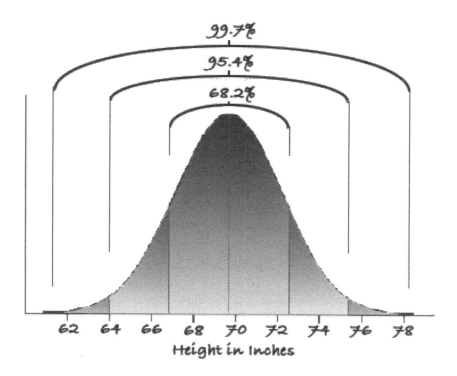

Ninety percent of twenty-five-year-old, white US men are between sixty-six inches (five feet six inches) and seventy-five inches
(six feet three inches), with the average and mean falling around
seventy inches (five feet ten inches). Five percent of men are
shorter than sixty-six inches, and another 5 percent of men are
taller than seventy-five inches. We call these men "outliers" on
the bell-shaped curve. Although most men are within four inches (two standard deviations) of the average, some men are not.
Similarly, although the average height is seventy inches, most
men are not exactly seventy inches tall. Almost half of American
men are a lot or a little shorter, and the other almost half are a
lot or a little taller.[13]

13 "National Center for Health Statistics," Centers for Disease Control and Prevention,
http://www.cdc.gov/nchs/fastats/body-measurements.htm. See Anthropometric Reference
Data for Children and Adults: United States, 2007–2010, table 12.

The same principle applies to blood-pressure statistics, cancer statistics, AIDS-survival statistics, and most other health measures. There are always outliers. A doctor may say people with a particular stage of a particular type of cancer have a survival rate of one to two years if they take a particular treatment. What the doctor is referring to is data that fall along a bell-shaped curve. So 90 percent of those patients live within two standard deviations of one to two years. But 5 percent live significantly longer, and 5 percent die much sooner. There is no harm in aiming to fit in with the almost 50 percent who live at least a little longer than average or the 5 percent who live significantly longer than average, is there?

In addition, doctors quote published data that by their very nature, given the rapid pace of medical advances, are old news. Data published this year were probably collected a few years earlier. In the interim, new treatments and new ways of combining old treatments are likely to have been developed. Interpreting a doctor's statement about prognosis as a factual prediction is an error. At best it is an educated guess.

It is inaccurate to say that most twenty-five-year-old, white, American men are seventy inches tall, even though that is the average height of such men in the United States. Similarly, it is inaccurate to say that, because the average survival with a particular illness is one year, your loved one's survival will be one year. Statements of prognosis are based on averages and do not truly predict where an individual will fall on the broad spectrum of possibilities. There are so many factors, known and unknown, that influence prognosis. Having tall parents, good nutrition, and a normal gestation will make it more likely that an individual American male will be taller than average. Having a healthy lifestyle, no other medical problems, and access to excellent medical care will increase the likelihood of a longer-than-average survival.

One of Bill's oncologists offered us a useful metaphor. He said, "All we need is the next piece of pavement for you to put your foot down on. We don't need the whole highway yet."

This gave us a nice image of workers diligently laying out the street in front of us. As long as our pace didn't exceed theirs, we would continue to have a place to go. Even if a cure wasn't found for Bill's illness during his lifetime, we hoped scientific research and trials would outpace us just enough to keep his disease from getting worse.

Sometimes I feel inclined to suppress positive thoughts. But I know rationally that being positive isn't going to keep the medicine from working (just like those thoughts won't cause it to work, either). It's such a warped idea that we can jinx something good just by our thoughts—that by feeling happy about something, we will make it go away.

Denial Versus Reality

It's not denial. I'm just selective about the reality I accept.
—BILL WATTERSON (*CALVIN AND HOBBES*)

When I talk to people, there sometimes seems to be this underlying or implicit inference like, "We know that Bill is choosing to delude himself and not face the facts, but how can you (a more practical person) deny what is really going on here?"

A few people confided in me their concern that Bill was in denial about his illness, implying I should do something to bring him to his senses. The word *denial* felt condemning, and this characterization bothered me. What exactly was he accused of denying? He knew he had cancer. He knew he was facing a tough battle. He knew the odds were stacked against him. However, he was choosing not to focus on any of that but instead to live in the present and to be hopeful.

Another articulated observation was the one that Bill was not being "realistic" about his diagnosis. Some people posed this as a deficiency that needed correction. But from my point of view, it wasn't as though I was in possession of the truth about what was to become of him so that I could set him straight. Instead, Bill and I chose to be skeptics of the idea that there was a specific reality to which we should simply subscribe. None of us knows what the future will bring.

Coming to terms with illness can be handled in dozens of ways, none more valid than the next. There were a few people who wanted Bill to react a certain way, and I had to discount their desires in favor of his. There were even a couple of times when I found myself intervening because I felt that Bill's best interests had a higher priority than someone else's agenda to force a certain perspective or degree of acceptance on him.

Rather than look at whether certain beliefs or thoughts are true, consider assessing whether they are helpful and useful.

Even in a case where someone appears to be losing the battle, is it really necessary for her to acknowledge that? What is wrong with a person taking her last breath thinking she is going to get better? Is that so terrible?

> Some may challenge your hopefulness, calling it denial. Denial, a defense against intolerable or too-intense feelings, is a psychological coping mechanism that serves a useful purpose. Sometimes bad news is too much to bear and overwhelms the recipient with negative emotion. Denial may serve as a temporary firewall, erected until the individual is able to process the information and attendant emotions. A classic example of denial is a person's initial response to hearing that someone has died unexpectedly. The first word out of that person's mouth is usually, "No!" When first given a bad diagnosis by a doctor, a patient will often ask, "Couldn't it just be…" This reflects an understandable wish to have the diagnosis be something less severe.

So long as denial does not interfere with the ability to respond appropriately to the challenge at hand, it need not be a problem. A woman who ignores a growing, ulcerating mass on her breast for months is in an unhealthy state of denial. A woman who refuses to say the word *cancer* but goes to the doctor and engages in the recommended treatment plan is doing what she needs to do to preserve her equanimity. She should not be forced to say the word *cancer*, because her denial is not interfering with her functioning.

Biologists have categorized three types of membranes: permeable, impermeable, and semipermeable. A permeable membrane permits substances to cross it freely, much as a sieve allows water to flow easily through. An impermeable membrane is a barrier that blocks virtually all flow from one side to the other; for example, the skull serves as an impermeable membrane between the brain and the scalp. A semipermeable membrane permits some substances to pass through but blocks others. The intestinal lining allows water and digested nutrients to cross into the bloodstream but blocks the passage of larger undigested material.

Our psychological defenses serve as a sort of semipermeable membrane between conscious awareness and the unconscious. They permit some information to freely cross into consciousness while other, potentially harmful information is held at bay. Denial is one of the densest fabrics in this membrane, but it will often loosen when the person is able to assimilate and digest difficult information. If a well-meaning person tells you that you or your loved one are in denial, tell that person that you or your loved one are doing the best you can to cope with the situation and that pushing you farther than you are ready to go will not help.

It is not always true that confronting reality is helpful or necessary. *Confront* is an aggressive word; it implies defiance, hostility, even battle. Do we really want to engage in a battle with a person who is coping with a life-threatening illness? Some people are not ready or able to "say goodbye," a concept that has been deemed important in contemporary death psychology. It is important to respect people's different preferences and capacities. Perhaps saying goodbye is not as important to someone as maintaining a peaceful spirit.

Pity and Self-Pity

Pity may represent little more than the impersonal concern which prompts the mailing of a check, but true sympathy is the personal concern which demands the giving of one's soul.
—Martin Luther King, Jr.

When people approach me with that poor-you look, I am forced to brace myself for some version of "It's so awful and sad what has happened to you." I freeze and hesitate at the simple question, "How are you?" I sink and quiver as I decide how to answer.

I get knowing looks, sad little nods. If I try to be positive, some people will humor me, but many look at me like I'm pathetically delusional.

Although I didn't have control over it, I felt extremely awkward when people treated us like we were characters in a tragic drama. I didn't like being the object of doleful looks and apprehensive approaches. I could sense the whispers of recognition: "She's the one who…"

It was a challenge to handle the frequently asked "How *are* you?" I never got comfortable with being the one everybody felt sorry for. Though friends always meant well when they asked about our well-being or the latest developments, I began to feel like I was walking around with a spotlight on me. I also felt as though I personified people's worst nightmares, and as the embodiment of their greatest fears, I found that some acquaintances approached me gingerly, as though I were carrying a potentially communicable plague. Some even avoided me altogether.

These interactions can be stressful on both sides, and as we discuss in chapter 4, I found it necessary to put thoughtful consideration into how much I exposed my emotions and to whom. It was helpful to me to have ready answers for inquiries about how we were doing so that I didn't have to struggle to answer very basic questions about Bill's condition and our family's well-being.

> There is a difference between empathy, sympathy, and pity. Empathy is the ability to feel what another person is feeling. An empathic listener, for example, might well up with tears when hearing a sad story told with feeling. The tired phrase "I feel your pain" has become a popular but perhaps insincere version of empathy. When we are the recipients of genuine empathy, we usually feel deeply understood and supported.
>
> Sympathy is the expression of sorrow at another person's misfortune. One can have sympathy for another person's suffering without necessarily feeling his or her pain. When we receive another person's sympathy, we may feel understood and supported, but perhaps less deeply than with empathy.
>
> Pity also involves sorrow or compassion for another person's misfortune but without the heartfelt identification with that person's situation. There is something about being the object of another person's pity that feels uncomfortable, like you are somehow diminished by your misfortune. "Oh, you poor thing" expresses pity but is not necessarily a comforting phrase.

When it came to self-pity, as much as I tried to avoid it, there certainly were occasions when I couldn't help but feel bad for Bill, our kids, and myself. I think it is only human to experience this state, because sometimes you just can't transcend the misery you feel for yourself. When this happened to me, I surrendered to those feelings and allowed myself to wallow in full-blown self-pity. But I tried not to get caught up there too long or too often, as a prolonged focus on my misfortune had the potential of being debilitating and incapacitating.

Another strategy is to just sit and let those thoughts and emotions wash over you and then watch them float away, not allowing them to take hold of your psyche or spirit. Some therapists describe this technique as similar to observing the traffic outside your window or clouds moving in the sky—notice them, sense them, but don't ascribe any particular meaning or importance to them. Sometimes it is helpful to simply accept our emotions and try not to allow them to paralyze or control us.

A companion to self-pity is what many feel as an overwhelming sense of unfairness. As much as we may object to situations that lack justice or reason, we have to acknowledge that the concept of fairness just doesn't apply to those out-of-our-control circumstances that befall us in real life. And even if we tried to analyze our lives in that light, it would only be fair to consider the positive as well as the negative.

I read somewhere about a woman who was terminally ill. Her daughter told her mother with admiration how amazing it was that she never said, "Why me?"

Her mother answered, "I never said 'why me' when all the good things in my life were happening; why would I say it now?"

> Self-pity was addressed by the great American playwright Edward Albee during an interview by Jesse Green for the *New York Times*. Albee said of the grief he felt when his partner of thirty-five years died of bladder cancer in 2005, "One thing I learned is that grief is easily turned into self-pity. Yes, someone you're with is fading, going out of focus." Albee cautions us not to lose sight of the fact that the person fighting illness has the greater loss. He reminds us that, "You can't just say, 'How dare you go away from me?'" He continues, "There's got to be a lot of, 'Thank you,' too. 'Thank you for being alive and being with me for so long.'" [14]

---

14 Jesse Greene, "Albee the Enigma, Now the Inescapable," *New York Times* (11 November 2007).

Albee's description suggests that grief is a paradox in which sorrow and gratitude take turns being figure and ground. This image of shifting the figure from sadness or self-pity about what you are going through now to gratitude for what you have been able to share with the person you love may be a helpful visual reminder to adjust your attitude when it gets stuck in self-pity.

Figure-Ground Illusion

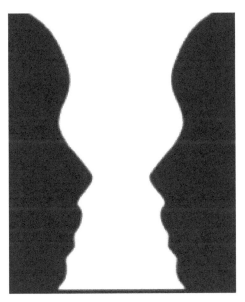

Cup or Faces Paradox (image created by Bryan Derksen.)[15]

A visual version of a paradox is the figure-ground illusion used by psychologists in the study of perception. In the illustration, most people first see a vase in the center of the picture and then observe the pair of faces looking toward each other. Once you see both, it is easy to shift your focus from one element of the illustration to the other.

15 Bryan Derksen, Cups or Faces Paradox. https://commons.wikimedia.org/wiki/File:Cup_or_faces_paradox.svg

The Virtue and Burden of Being Strong

> *You never know how strong you are until*
> *being strong is your only choice.*
> —Bob Marley

When we hold everything together while dealing with our loved one's illness or disability, we may find ourselves receiving praise and positive reinforcement for being "strong." While this is typically considered in our culture to be an admirable trait, it may backfire when taken to an extreme. What does it mean to be strong? Does it mean to soldier through all of life's challenges without emoting or faltering? Or does it mean to be in touch with our true authentic selves, even if that may reveal vulnerability or insecurity? Being the "strong one" can help us cope well with crisis. But at the same time, the struggle to maintain that position of strength may come at a cost. We may find ourselves detaching from our inner selves in order to fulfill the burden of living up to this standard, whether self-imposed or other-imposed. Maybe this is necessary for the short term, but at some point we all must connect with what is going on inside.

Perhaps it is helpful to think of other definitions for strength besides the usual concepts of power and indestructibility. Maybe it is strong to be honest, even if that means admitting our fatigue and fear. Or might we consider ourselves to be strong when we acknowledge that we are merely human, that we need help, or that we are overwhelmed? Hemingway wrote, "Many of us are strong in the broken places." Most people will find that both strength and vulnerability are companions to us on this ever-evolving journey.

There are times when being told how extraordinary one is can feel like an added burden. In Marge Piercy's poem, "For Strong Women," she expresses the loneliness of being told by others, "You're so strong." Being admired for your strength can create a feeling of isolation, as if you are doing all the heavy lifting while others stand aside and watch. It also may imply an expectation that you are so strong that you don't need any help. Piercy expresses the yearning we have to be recognized and loved for our vulner-abilities as well as our strengths. Deeming someone strong with-out validating the personal struggles that developed that person's strength diminishes the person's whole experience. Pointing to the importance of our interconnectedness, she concludes, "Until we are all strong together, a strong woman is a woman strongly afraid."[16] It is important to ask for acknowledgment, to have a wit-ness when that is what you want, but also to be able to ask for help when you need another person to roll up his or her sleeves and pull alongside you.

The Power of Language

Words are but the signs of ideas.
—Samuel Johnson

Words are persuasive, and as I began to discover their power, I became more deliberate about their selection. One day when Bill was in active treatment, he asked me, "At what point can we use the term *survivor*?" He was concerned that he didn't technically qualify for the label, since he still had cancer and didn't know whether he would, indeed, survive the illness. My instinct was to answer, "Now." He was surviving it now, so he was a survivor.

You may become aware of how your choice of words reflects your attitude. Do you think of your loved one as "living with" or "dying from" his or her illness? Many people tend to look at illness in clear-cut terms. They believe a person is either cured of or dies from his or her condition. But the reality is that, for many people, even very serious illnesses can be man-aged as chronic diseases. Often, when cancer can't be cured, it can at least be maintained for many, many years, just like diabetes. Our perspective can affect and, in turn, be affected by the phrases we use. Is your loved one a victim or a survivor?

---

16 Marge Piercy, *The Moon Is Always Female* (New York: Alfred Knopf, 1986), 56.

And can we go even further? I recently spoke with a woman who is living with a serious mental illness. She told me that being a "survivor" does not feel like much of an accomplishment to her, given the challenges she faces on a daily basis. She prefers to think of herself as a "thriver." Whichever one prefers, I believe both terms can give a person a great deal of pride and comfort. It is more than a description of a person's health; it is a state of mind. I have never met anyone who has been helped by viewing himself or herself as a "cancer victim."

Our own words can affect our loved one's perception: "You are living with cancer." "You are living with AIDS." "You are living with hepatitis." Not dying from it—as long as you're alive, you are living with it.

Having spent the past twenty-five years working in some aspect of health care, I have noticed a shift in focus and the accompanying vernacular to concentrate more on *health* and less on *illness*. In an effort to empower people and make them more responsible for their physical and mental conditions, medical clinics see the wisdom of addressing *wellness*, including smoking cessation, weight control, addiction treatment, and stress reduction. It is not uncommon to hear a physician recommend yoga or holistic remedies to patients to help with healing of the mind, body, and spirit.

Even when illnesses appear to have attacked randomly and with no regard for our health choices and behavior, our attitudes toward these conditions can have a big impact on how we perceive the role they have in our overall lives. And the language we choose in describing them only reinforces those attitudes for better or worse.

> Thoughts and feelings shape our language, and language shapes our thoughts and feelings. If our thoughts or our feelings are depressed, we will tend to say pessimistic or depressed things. Conversely, if we choose negative themes in our language, our thoughts and feelings are likely to become more depressed. This

is the essential premise behind cognitive therapy for depression, a treatment developed by Aaron Beck, MD.[17]

Cognitive therapy aims to identify and correct dysfunctional thoughts, such as "I always mess things up. There's really no point in trying." A thought like that leads to feeling ineffective and hopeless. A corrected thought might be "I messed this up when I tried it last time, but maybe if I try it a different way, I'll be more successful." These words lead to a greater sense of efficacy and hope.

If you choose pessimistic language about your loved one's illness, you are likely to feel depressed and demoralized. The statement "I cannot cope with my mother's dementia" is not likely to lead to thoughts or feelings that help you cope. On the other hand, a statement like "I am overwhelmed by my mother's dementia; maybe I should talk to someone to get some practical advice about how to proceed" leads to a feeling of hope and a plan about how to get help and feel better.

When We Become the Illness

Reality doesn't bite; rather, our perception of reality bites.
—ANTHONY J. D'ANGELO

Often when we learn about our loved one's serious diagnosis, we let our lives become primarily about that illness or disability, leading us into a detrimental trap. We may also find that others begin to define our loved one by his illness, identifying the ways he is different or disabled and making assumptions about his functionality, longevity, and ability. Likewise, the

---

17 Aaron T. Beck, A. John Rush, Brian F. Shaw, and Gary Emery, *Cognitive Therapy of Depression* (New York: Guilford Press, 1979).

person with the illness or disability may begin to overly self-identify with the condition. She may park in a disabled parking spot when she doesn't really need to, complain in detail about her discomforts, or play the cancer card.

There are times, of course, when the illness card can be an expedient obstruction to people who attempt to engage you in things you just can't make a priority. For example, shortly after Bill was diagnosed, someone I barely knew called me about a minor playground issue that had taken place at the elementary school and didn't directly involve my child. When she started to go into all the details, I just had to cut her off. Maybe it was harsh of me, but I said, "I'm sorry, but my husband has just been diagnosed with cancer. I can't deal with that right now."

I imagine she was stunned (although, amazingly, it didn't stop her from calling me a week later to resume her concern), but I decided I had the right to be honest about where my priorities were. Maybe I gave myself a little extra permission to be blunter than I usually am in an effort to protect myself from her officiousness.

However, there is a danger that by habitually using the illness as a shield, we may lose sight of all our other qualities and capabilities, making our lives only or overwhelmingly about the illness or disability. It also allows the illness to become all-powerful, which is exactly what we want to avoid. With the illness already grabbing a substantial piece of our lives, we want to refrain from encouraging it to consume an even larger share.

The tendency to narrow our thinking about our loved one can also extend to the way we think about ourselves as family members. In devoting so much of our time, energy, and thoughts to our loved one's illness, we can become mired in that role. By excessively focusing on our identities as caregivers, as spouses, parents, or children of someone who is sick or disabled, we can neglect other aspects of our lives, missing out on roles and activities in which we might also find purpose and passion.

When Bill was first diagnosed, I felt like I became a new person. In a matter of seconds, I turned into a woman whose husband had cancer. That new identity was first and foremost in my mind at all times. Everything I thought or did was impacted by my revised self-perception. It took a very conscious effort for me to reintegrate all the other pieces of me that were still relevant and vital. I learned to realize that, despite this turn of events, it was important not to lose sight of the fact that I was still me.

The words we use to describe ourselves are meaningful, and the way we choose to say things can have a significant impact on how we think and feel. For example, mental-health advocates have worked for decades to get physicians and policy makers to call people with schizophrenia just that rather than "schizophrenics." The difference, although superficially subtle, is profound. A person with schizophrenia is first a person and, as a person, deserves to be treated with the same respect and dignity as any other person. The phrase "with schizophrenia" is merely a modifier, describing one aspect of the person. Calling someone a "schizophrenic" reduces that person's identity to the psychiatric diagnosis and has a dehumanizing effect on the individual and for treatment planners and policy makers.

Similarly, saying "a person fighting cancer" or "a person living with MS" leaves room for that person to also have other characteristics, whereas "a cancer patient" restricts the person's identity to a single diagnosis. This phenomenon has been widely observed among people with HIV infection. When people say, "I'm HIV," rather than, "I have HIV," their identity and existence shrinks down to a tiny, viral particle, and they lose themselves in this self-definition.

Psychologically defining one's self by the diagnosis paves the way to being ruled by the illness. It is more adaptive to establish an identity that includes the diagnosis in a long list of other attributes that also describe the person, such as "a married, forty-five-year-old mother of two teenagers, who works part-time as an accountant, makes jewelry in her spare time, and just learned she has cervical cancer." Such a self-definition permits the speaker and the listener to appreciate the multiple roles this woman has in her life; "cancer patient" is only one part of her existence. She is more likely to make cancer treatment fit into her life if she defines herself also as a wife, mother, worker, and jewelry designer. Reducing herself to merely a "cancer patient" opens the door to losing her sense of identity, abandoning her hobby, and placing everything on hold. That is an implicit invitation to the cancer to take over her life.

Being Flexible and Resilient

> *Adapt or perish, now as ever, is*
> *nature's inexorable imperative.*
> —H. G. WELLS

I remember first really understanding the idea of flexibility when I became a parent. Bill and I had been leading a busy social life, and we expected our newborn child to fit right into it. Fortunately for us, our daughter was an easygoing baby whom we could readily schlepp to anything that was on our calendars. She slept through movies and dinners out. She cooed and flirted at parties. She even played quietly on a blanket on the floor for hours at my office.

Then one night the three of us were all dressed up and about to go to a function. Our daughter threw up all over herself and me. That was the end of our evening out. We had a sick baby, not to mention that our nicest outfits were out of commission. For a little while, I was disappointed. I wasn't used to someone else altering my plans. But I realized how lucky I was to have this darling baby who was only temporarily ill. And so began a more mature perspective that my life wasn't all about me. I acclimated to being accommodating and learned to adjust to those last-minute changes that happen to everyone but are compounded when you integrate multiple people into your life. I appreciated that I had people whom I loved in my life, even if they did sometimes ruin my plans.

Adapting to change, as mundane as a spoiled evening out or as monumental as a grim medical diagnosis, is a skill that can be cultivated and honed.

As life changes from its expected course, we must learn to adapt. Dealing with a significant medical condition entails doctor's appointments, treatments, visitors, and disruptions in work and home schedules. We become more flexible in order to make everything fit. Like a San Francisco skyscraper designed to sway in a quake, we, too, have to learn to absorb and bow with our personal shock waves.

It can be helpful to choose an attribute you most want for yourself and have that be your watchword as you move through the process. This happened for me one afternoon when I was at a school event with my daughter. As an icebreaker, we were each instructed to design a name tag with our first name and an adjective that described us. It was intended to be an aspirational adjective, a quality we hoped would define us. This was a month or two after Bill's diagnosis, and my self-perception felt rather shaky and amorphous. How would I describe myself? How would I *like* to describe myself? Hopeful? Persistent? Functioning? Finally I came up with "resilient." That was the attribute I most hoped to cultivate.

In the few minutes allotted to us to decorate our name tags, I pondered this adjective. I wanted to figure out how to enhance my inner character strengths that would allow me to bounce back after each adversity in my life, big or small. I hoped to be a person who would not be defeated by difficult life circumstances. I longed to learn these skills so that I might teach them to my children. Emotional resilience seemed like a good goal for me, because ideally it would be independent of whatever life events would actually occur.

In the months that followed, I attempted to foster this attribute by looking for my own role models of resilience. Some were very proximate—members of my immediate family, living and dead. Some were public figures, current or in history. Some were even anecdotal—people I had heard of, friends of friends. This cast of allies helped me nurture the idea that if they could do it, so could I.

CHAPTER 3
Walking the Path

As you adjust to your loved one's illness, it is helpful to find a balance between making room for what must be done to care for him or her and holding on to what gives your life rhythm and meaning. In this chapter, we discuss strategies for finding that balance, which include accepting that change is necessary, controlling worry, correcting dysfunctional thought patterns, and practicing mindfulness.

A New Normal

> *Time is a dressmaker specializing in alterations.*
> —Faith Baldwin

> *This weekend has been very low-key. We canceled all of our plans and just spent time together as a family. I know we can't—and it wouldn't be healthy to—do this only and always, but this narrowing in feels so good. I have more anxiety about Bill when we're apart. He feels less tangible, like he could be lost. But as C said, "This was not a plane crash." Bill is still here. I need to be here, too.*

One thing I noticed in the first few weeks and months after Bill was diagnosed was that I suffered a fair amount of separation anxiety when I was away from him. When we were together and I could see him, touch him, and talk to him, I could relax. In a strange, irrational way, I think I considered myself to be sort of an amulet, such that as long as I was with him, nothing bad could happen. But when we were both at our respective offices or when, on occasion, one of us was out of town, I would feel anxious that I wasn't with him to see that he was OK, to protect him. I found myself checking in with him many times a day just to hear his voice.

I felt most secure in the evenings when, after the kids were in bed, we would lie side by side on the couch and I would put my ear on his chest. I needed to hear his heart beating. I needed to hear him breathe. I would listen to his bad lung—it sounded fine to me. How could he be so sick? We had whole conversations with my continuing in this position, listening to his voice through his chest. If only I could stay with him all the time, I could make sure his heart was still beating; I could make sure he was drawing breaths from both of his lungs.

As Bill began his treatment, we imagined a little chemo brigade marching through his body, stalking and trapping the bad cells and then annihilating them with relentless precision. Whatever the costs would be—loss of hair, energy, appetite—we would happily pay them in return for success on the battlefield. We approached the fight with determination, with hope that our weapons would prove to be sufficiently potent.

But even so, we recognized that the battle we were fighting while continuing to live our preexisting lives was our new normal. As much as this disease and its impact on everything felt like an unacceptable intrusion into our lives, we had to cope with the fact that it was likely here to stay.

> Interweave your old ways of being together with your new reality in order to maintain a thread of continuity in your relationship. Some people are so frightened by illness that they freeze in its presence. They may feel as if their loved one has suddenly become a stranger, and they're not sure how to behave. Little rituals that have always existed between you should be continued, perhaps in a modified form if need be.

If a married couple always shared a cup of coffee together in the morning, but now her medical condition precludes coffee, share a glass of juice instead so that the morning time together is preserved. If you and your sister loved to exchange irreverent jokes, don't stop them just because she's ill. Her wicked sense of humor is one of her best allies and will reinforce the bond between you during this difficult time.

Particularly with injuries and illnesses that create a disfigurement, such as a severe burn or a mastectomy, people bearing the illness may feel embarrassed or ashamed of how they look. This can affect their willingness to go out in public, and it can cause inhibition in intimate relationships. If your loved one has these feelings, offer reassurance, not just in your words but through your behavior. The wife of one of my patients had a mastectomy to treat breast cancer, and this took a terrible toll on her self-image. By holding her, caressing her, and demonstrating that he was not afraid of or repulsed by her scar, her husband helped her heal the internal wound caused by the external one.

This *Is* Your Life

> *[If] there is a sin against life, it consists perhaps not so much in despairing of life as in hoping for another life and in eluding the implacable grandeur of this life.*
> —ALBERT CAMUS

This is my life. This is my life. This is my life. This is my life. This is my life.

Often, when our lives are not going the way we anticipated, we get into a mind-set that we just need to get through the rough spot before we return to the status quo to which we have become accustomed. We think we can just wait out the limbo. When we have an exam or a work deadline looming, we may coach ourselves to rally to a level of high performance that involves long hours, little sleep, and rigorous intellectual effort, knowing that this surge will be time limited. But in the case of illness, we need to accept that the departure from our comfortable routine may be long-term or even permanent; we have embarked on a new course.

I remember one day going to see my therapist when I was eager to share how inspired I had been by a bumper sticker I had recently seen. "Happiness is enjoying the detours of life," I repeated to her.

She thought about this and helped me see that this *is* my life, not a detour. She even drew a picture, giving me a helpful visual (figure A). I was seeing my life as a straight line, and then there was an abrupt turn that was the detour. Instead, she drew a straight line that was interrupted by a blockade that said, "No longer an option." At that point, there was a turn, and this was the direction my life took. Not a detour, but my actual life.

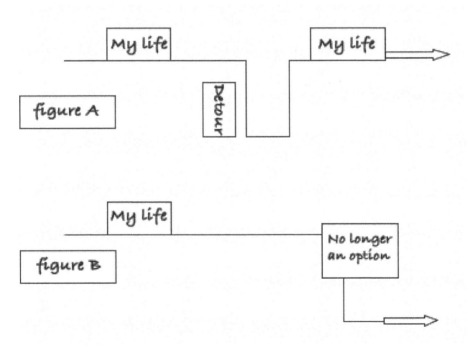

It was vital for me to understand that the road I was traveling was my road, however unexpected or undesired. It wasn't merely a brief bypass that would return me to my regular life. No matter the eventual outcome, I was now on a new path that was my real life, bumps and all. Even if Bill's illness were to be successfully treated, I would be a changed person simply from going through this experience.

As is often said, only our expectations can cause us disappointment. In order to cope with the turn in the road, we may need to revise our assumptions. If we move through our lives with hard and fast expectations, we can have a lifetime of disappointments. So many things can intervene in our journey or disrupt our carefully laid plans. The better we can experience the present without an eye toward an expectation that may or may not happen, the less likely we are to be disappointed when our route is redirected.

At times I was convinced I would wake up and realize this turn of events was just a bad dream. We all have those middle-of-the-night jolts when we startle awake and realize, with instant gratitude, that a dreadful and seemingly real scenario was only a nightmare. In the early days and weeks, I found myself waiting to be so awakened in relief. There were times in the groggy, opening seconds of morning when I would bask in the momentary shelter of innocence. Then, suddenly, the horror of Bill's diagnosis would flood my mind as though I were discovering it for the first time.

At another time in my life, during a happy transition, I had experienced the same morning phenomenon. Those first few mornings after our eldest child was born, I would awaken to the newborn cry. *Oh, yeah, I have a baby!* I would realize, jumping out of bed. I was a different person now: I was a mother. I was filled with anticipation and joy.

Later, in a similar but sad way, I would shudder several seconds into my day, *Oh, yeah, my husband has cancer.* Again I was a different person. I was a young wife and mother whose husband had a grave illness. Now it wasn't as easy to jump out of bed. My desire was to pull the covers over my head and try again for another, better wakening thought. But of course this thought was the truth, my life.

And it was my job to get up and live it.

> Although a lot of medical disorders have a clear beginning and end, others become chronic problems that require long-term management. When an injury first occurs or an illness manifests its first symptoms, we naturally set out to diagnose and fix the problem. We have expectations about the time needed for recovery: we may give influenza one week, a broken bone six weeks, recovery from thoracic surgery two months, recovery from an episode of major depression three to six months, and treatment of cancer one to two years. But it may take a person longer to fully recover from any of these, or a full recovery may not occur, in which case the person is left with a chronic illness.

> At some point, the person with the illness and his family and friends begin to realize that the illness is not merely a visitor but has come to stay. This process of realization is often accompanied by grief, including the anger and sadness that are part of the grief response.

> I recall a conversation with a mother who had first sought mental-health treatment for her daughter when the girl was in fifth grade. The child was sullen, did not play or interact much with her classmates, and had violent temper tantrums at home. For the first year or two, the parents took their daughter to several child psychiatrists, got psychological testing, engaged in family therapy in addition to individual therapy for their daughter, and tried a series of medications. They maintained great hope, believing that if they tried hard and found the right combination of treatments, they would be able to recapture their dream of a "normal" daughter who would grow up, go to college, and have a happy life.

By the time their daughter was in eighth grade, they had given up hope of a cure. They shifted their efforts to finding a therapeutic high-school environment and a behavior therapist who would help their daughter learn and practice appropriate life skills, such as effectively asking for what she wants, managing interpersonal conflict, and reducing stress.

The process of shifting expectations was very painful for the parents. Although they had tried everything, they still worried that they were giving up prematurely. They also felt angry with medical providers for failing to cure their daughter and with their daughter for not responding to treatment. Only by shifting their expectations could they make appropriate plans for their child, let go of their guilt and resentment, and focus instead on the positive aspects of their relationship.

Taking One Step at a Time

The secret of health for both mind and body is not to mourn for the past, worry about the future, or anticipate troubles, but to live in the present moment wisely and earnestly.
—BUDDHA

How do we get into a mental framework where we aren't just living from appointment to appointment? From test to test? Whether Bill has months or years, there will always be a next test for him. We have to learn to live fully in between the tests—otherwise we won't be able to get beyond a constant state of anxiety. I need to get into the frame of mind where the next thing is something good and soon and normal. Instead of thinking about the next test, I need to think about the next dinner I will prepare for the family tonight or next week when we go to the mountains for spring break.

The idea of living in the present is so much the foundation of every self-help book that it has become a cliché. There is nothing original about the pearl of wisdom that we need to live mindfully in the present. But this cliché is true. The present is all we have. All of us.

When my children were in preschool, I noticed over and over again how a roomful of tiny people had the natural instinct to live in the moment. Until they were constantly drilled to *hurry, hurry, hurry* to the next thing, their innate tendency was to just be. But after years of "We need to go," "We're late," and "We'll miss out," kids become accustomed to the urgency we have trained them to incorporate into their psyches. The future is more important than the now.

What a disservice we do by imposing our anxious projections on their instinctive abilities to live in the present. As a parent of young children, I came to appreciate how their emotions were so much less complicated than mine, because they were not accompanied by hand-wringing about the past and anxiety about the future. A five-year-old's emotional state can change in an instant; it doesn't incorporate the deeply rooted, baggage-laden burdens we adults carry.

When we spend time in the past or in the future, we are robbing ourselves of our ability to rally our mental resources around matters of the present. By staying in the now, we give our energy to that which is currently on our plate without obsessing over what we already ate or may need to bite off later.

> *I have to integrate the belief that whatever happens, I will be able to handle it. But I only need to handle whatever is right in front of me, like putting a smile on my face in a few minutes when I go pick up the kids. On Wednesday, I will need to handle the appointment with the doctor. On Thursday, I will need to handle any postchemo reaction Bill might have. But he also might not have any reactions, and then I won't have to handle that.*

It can be completely overwhelming when you let it sink in how much life has changed and will continue to change. I would frequently wonder how I was going to do everything that would be required of me.

When an appointment was imminent, I would fret not only about what we would find out but also about everything else that would happen after that. So I would start with worrying about what might happen at the appointment tomorrow and what the CAT scan would show *and*, if it was bad, what treatment might Bill be offered *and*, if he received the treatment, whether it would be successful *and*, if it wasn't successful, how we would handle it *and* whether there would be any more treatments available *and* whether they would be successful, and on and on. I was capable of going way down the road in my head.

Conjuring up a mental avalanche wasn't useful for me. As boulders engulfed my consciousness, I would lose sight of the one thing that actually needed my immediate attention. Extricating myself from the multitude of thoughts was critical to preventing self-suffocation.

Sometimes, when my mind was racing so fast and I felt I was projecting unproductively and obsessively into the future, I would muster up a stern but compassionate internal voice. "Stop it, Laura," I would say to myself. "Take a deep breath and stop the ruminating. This isn't helpful." And then I would try to distract myself with another topic, just as I might redirect a child to a better, safer toy.

Negative thinking is common for most people, especially when we are overwhelmed. Replacing those thoughts with more positive ones can make a huge difference. Repeating a comforting affirmation like a mantra is a productive strategy for many people. Here are a few to try:

- "I have handled this before; I can handle it again."
- "I will learn from this, and it will be easier next time."
- "It's OK to feel angry/sad/frustrated sometimes."
- "I shouldn't be disappointed at myself when I feel overwhelmed. I am human."
- "I am resilient. I am a survivor."

Today we had the distressing news we were dreading. The first round of chemo didn't work, and we're on to plan B. People say, "You'll deal with the information when you get it," and of course that's true. You don't have a choice. No amount of fretting or obsessing changed one iota the information we got today and the fact that we had to process and deal with it on the spot.

This skill of dealing only with what was before me at the moment was totally contrary to my nature. The only way I could manage was by breaking down the seemingly huge scenario into small, manageable parts and tackling them one at a time.

I would say to myself, "Today we will see the doctor, and I can do that. Tomorrow we will get the test results, and I will deal with that information when we get it. All I need to do is get through today. Tomorrow I'll get through tomorrow. Next week I'll deal with next week."

Gradually I was able to take each step as I needed to: "Today, I need to get his medications, and I can do that." "Today I need to write the appeal to the insurance company, and I can do that." "Today I need to take him for his surgery, and I can do that."

And sometimes, if it was a task that could wait, I gave myself permission to say, "Actually, I can't do that today."

The Buddhist teaching to live in the present moment—being fully aware of what is happening now rather than dwelling on the past or worrying about the future—is becoming a familiar idea in modern society. Staying focused on the reality at hand helps you respond appropriately and helpfully. There are several techniques to help foster the ability to stay focused on the present, also called "mindfulness."

The most common technique is meditation, in which one sits quietly and clears the mind. There are many techniques for meditation. One involves focusing on a repeated phrase or mantra. Another empties the mind by focusing on the breath. A third listens nonjudgmentally to the thoughts running through one's head without letting one's attention get attached to the thoughts. With any of these three techniques, thoughts will enter the mind; rather than focusing on any particular thought, the trick is to let the thoughts travel by.

A helpful visualization is to consider your thoughts a river and see yourself sitting on the bank of the river, watching all those thoughts go by. If you latch on to a thought, you will find yourself in the water, swept along by the current. As soon as you become aware of this, get out of the river and sit peacefully on the bank once more. With practice, people who meditate become aware that worries are products of the mind and that they can choose to let them go by shifting their focus. There are an abundance of guided meditation apps and audio files available online for free or for a small fee. These provide an easy entry into meditation for the novice.

In an attempt to localize the areas of the brain affected by meditation practice, Western scientists have studied brain changes in people who meditate. So far each study has found a different area that is built up by meditation. What these areas have in common is that they are all involved in pathways that process emotional information.

Getting a Handle on Worrying

Worrying is like paying on a debt that may never come due.
—WILL ROGERS

As much as I knew rationally that worrying is not productive and doesn't change anything, sometimes it was impossible not to do so, especially when major test results were imminent. A chemotherapy trial Bill was in required that he have a CAT scan or X-ray every three weeks before he received his next treatment. I learned to train myself not to start my worrying until a day or two before the test. My most relaxed time was after a treatment, when I would have another three-week interval before the next test and could postpone my worrying again. It was like the stress that builds up before a work deadline or an exam. As soon as it was over, there was a lightening of the burden before it began to escalate again.

I have an acquaintance whose son was diagnosed with a very aggressive, fast-growing tumor. Although it was successfully removed, it has a 40 percent recurrence rate. This boy must have labs drawn every quarter to make sure he is clean of any cancerous cells. His mother commented to me that every three months, right before he is due for these tests, she starts to think about it. The rest of the time, she puts it out of her mind. It is the way she copes.

Think about other times in your life when you have had a big worry but somehow learned to manage it. For example, when your teenager gets his driver's license, you may obsess about fears every time he is on the road or the first time he takes the highway or drives in a storm or goes to the mountains. But at some point, you have to let go of the worry, even though it continues to be a potentially dangerous activity over which you have little control.

When our first child began to drive, we had done what we could to prepare. She had gone to an excellent driving school, had a safe car, and had been the recipient of every conceivable piece of parental automotive advice. She had a good head on her shoulders and had no history of being careless or reckless in any way. When, much to Bill's and my secret disappointment, she passed her driving exam on her sixteenth birthday, we were forced to send her, license in hand, out into the world of people in cars. There wasn't any more we could do. Worrying didn't accomplish anything, and making her call us every time she reached her destination became unreasonable. Ultimately we learned to manage our anxiety. In fact, we mastered it so well that very quickly we entrusted her with the lives of her younger siblings.

I have learned that it can be helpful to manage our health worries the same way. We do what we can. We research options; we find a doctor we trust; we ask questions; we comply perfectly with medical instructions.

Combining these taxing activities with ineffective worrying compounds our stress and is the opposite of helpful. At some point, we must trust that we are doing all we can do. Somehow we have to get the upper hand so that the fretting is managed in the same way that we handle other thoughts of hazard or harm.

> *This way that I mentally go through all of the what-ifs over and over comes from an illogical assumption that if I can think about everything that could possibly happen, then I will have no surprises. And I hate surprises.*

On several occasions, I received the advice "Hope for the best; prepare for the worst." For the most part, this was not a particularly valuable tip for me, especially since I already had an unhealthy tendency to obsessively mentally prepare for the worst. As we discuss in the next section, there are some productive preparations you can attempt, so it is important to sort those out from the useless, incessant worrying that can be mistaken for preparation. The reality is that no amount of worrying is going to serve as a preventive or immunizing tool.

When sitting in limbo, we may be inclined to ruminate over past events that we cannot change or project into the future, which we irrationally believe we can control with our thoughts. Our anxiety often manifests itself in relentless worrying. In my case, I found I could spend an excessive amount of time and energy worrying about things that might happen or might not happen. These thoughts plagued me during the day, kept me up at night, and even insinuated themselves into my dreams.

Eventually I realized I must have been getting something out of it or else I wouldn't do it so much. What was the benefit I was receiving? As irrational as it might sound, I must have believed that worrying would do one of two things: 1) prevent the thing I was worrying about from happening or 2) prepare me for the bad thing happening, thus making it easier if it did. My logical self knew that neither of those outcomes would be the result of my obsessive thoughts, but my unconscious self persisted in this behavior nonetheless.

When we allow our minds to become mired in anticipating future misery, we are in effect choosing current misery with the misconception that we might spare ourselves later. It is rather ironic that we create so much suffering in the present on the pretense that we are preventing it at a future date.

Using a trivial example: If I spend all week worrying that the predicted snowstorm on Friday will thwart people from coming to the big party I am planning, I am projecting that I will be unhappy if my party fails to meet my expectations. However, if I start to anticipate that unhappiness on Monday, I am adding a week of misery to the presumed misery that may or may not occur on Friday. Perhaps the weather won't be so bad, or perhaps people will venture out despite the cold. And if my fears are valid and I have a lot of food and no guests, I will deal with those logistics and feelings when and if they happen.

At some level, we believe our thoughts are very powerful. We are tricked into imagining that we may be able to control outcomes in the world merely by thinking in a certain way. A friend once told me a story about a relative who fretted about every possible calamity that might befall her children. She worried that they could be injured while skiing, that they might be in a bad car accident, that they would contract a terrible disease. She thought of almost every conceivable harm and thus in some way believed that her mental projections guaranteed the safety of her family. But this woman did not think to worry about her son getting attacked by a shark in Australia. Despite all that time spent worrying, her thoughts were not able to avert the tragic (and unimaginable) death of her beloved son.

The dilemma posed by worrying is that it presents us with both the desire for control as well as the discomfort of uncertainty. We are drawn toward control, even when we know it to be unattainable. We understand the reality of uncertainty, even when we resist surrendering to it.

It is often said, "Don't spend time crossing bridges you may never get to." There's a reason this adage is so overused: it is sage advice. It makes sense to stay on this side of the bridge, because it is neither helpful nor productive to imagine or fixate on the demons on the other side that you might not ever encounter. Don't let negative inner chatter envelop your consciousness; most of the things we worry about will never happen. Quieting the mind is not easy, but when we are able to do so, I am convinced we have a better quality of life. We are certainly not contributing positively to our psyches by preemptively snatching away what we value most.

In my case, I constantly wondered, *Will this be our last trip, our last Thanksgiving, our last whatever?* Not only did I inhibit my own enjoyment of special occasions, but I also lost sight of the fact that *no one* knows when our last anything will be. Even a death-row inmate eating what has been deemed his or her final meal can receive a last-minute stay of execution.

But there were times when every one of my strategies failed. Even as I tried blocking my natural inclination to project into the future, there were occasions when I just had to let my mind wander *there*—to what might happen. Sometimes we need to consider the worst-case scenario in order to determine if there are any practical things we need to do now or just because we can no longer resist the pull of particular thoughts that we have treated as forbidden.

Therefore, when it became too difficult or unreasonable to stifle every thought about the future, I would allow myself a limited amount of time to ponder the things I felt I needed to consider in order to have a tentative plan about what I might do *if*. In the case of thoughts that were practical and required attention (*What will happen to Bill's health insurance if he becomes too sick to work?*), I would put those follow-up items on my actual list of things to do. In the case of thoughts that were nagging at me but weren't productive (*What would I do if I were a widow?*), I would let myself think about them for a little while and then put those thoughts away.

A coping strategy I learned when Bill was sick is the container exercise. When thoughts feel overwhelming, it can be helpful to imagine a container with a lid—a plastic tub, a shoebox, a treasure chest, anything that suits your fancy—in which you can securely store difficult emotions and feelings. In my case, the visualization was simple but effective. I found a place in the top corner of my bedroom where I mentally installed an imaginary shelf. When I needed to consider my darkest thoughts, I allotted a few minutes and then imagined myself putting those thoughts in a box and placing it on my shelf. I am not a visual person, but even I was able to engage myself in this invented ritual when necessary. I would let my mind go there—to what might happen. But it was a finite and controlled process, not a psychological free-for-all. Putting my thoughts on paper was another way I regularly allowed the tough feelings to surface and attempted to work through them.

> While staying focused on the present is helpful for responding in a calm and effective manner, it is natural and adaptive to think about the future, too, in order to plan. Too much time thinking about the future might mean a person is worrying in an unproductive way, while no time thinking about the future may leave a person unprepared for change. As in most things, moderation is the key.

> A woman who takes care of her chronically ill husband may find herself worrying about whether they will be able to keep their house if he dies. It may not be appropriate or comfortable for her to share these fears with her husband, but it may be helpful for her to discuss them with a financial adviser or family member. A realistic and pragmatic plan about how she will survive financially may help her settle more comfortably into the present-day task of supporting her husband through his illness.

> Some people find it difficult to stop their worrying. They experience a seemingly endless cascade of fears and doubts. One approach to managing nonproductive worry is to compartmentalize both the content and duration of the worry. An example of compartmentalizing the content is "Today I will worry about how I will pay for the medical bills, but I won't worry about how to pay for the kids' college education, which I'll worry about another day."

An example of compartmentalizing duration is permitting yourself to worry for only ten minutes and enforcing that by setting a timer or permitting yourself to worry only during your morning walk. If a worry comes up later in the day, make a mental note to consider it on your next walk, and then put it out of your mind by changing the subject. This takes practice and discipline, but it is very effective.

If you find that after employing the strategies we discuss in this chapter, you still cannot get incessant worrying or obsessive thoughts under control, you might seek professional help through therapy or medications. We discuss psychiatric and psychological care in more detail in chapter 7.

When it comes to helping children who are close to the person with the illness, it is important to try as much as possible to alleviate their anxiety and burden. For Bill and me in our role as parents, our top priority was to try to spare our kids, as much as possible, from being constantly plagued by worries. So from the beginning, we told them we would take care of monitoring the situation so that they wouldn't need to spend time worrying. We said we would keep them informed if there were changes they should know about. I believe this relieved them of feeling the weight and fear of uncertainty to a large extent. While we couldn't promise them that nothing bad would happen, we assured them we would absorb the responsibility for staying vigilant about developments.

Refraining from Overgeneralizations

We are more prone to generalize the bad than the good.
We assume the bad is more potent and contagious.
—Georg Hegel

I have to regard the good moments and not-so-good moments just as they are: moments. Not as foretellers of what is to come. It's like I have to make a deal with myself not to let a bad appointment send me into despair but also not to let a good appointment get me too elated. Staying in the present goes both ways. Bad day, period. Good day, period. Bad appointment, period. Good appointment, period. Don't get carried away—in either direction.

A lesson that most of us try to teach our children from an early age is that they shouldn't be quick to assign labels to others or to their experiences. For example, just because a classmate may struggle in school, it does not mean that student is unintelligent. Just because a certain team lost a game, that doesn't mean the players are bad. And yet as adults, we frequently overgeneralize. One action can make a person completely incompetent or totally brilliant in our eyes. In dealing with Bill's illness, I had to become aware of my tendency to jump too hastily to large conclusions: His coughing more meant he was getting worse. His running faster meant he was getting better. I had to make a concerted effort to reel that in.

I found it useful to find value in something positive without projecting to an all-out cure or find disappointment in something negative without projecting to a huge turn for the worse. I attempted to do this by keeping my observations (whether good or bad) very limited: "Oh, he had a long workout; he seems to be feeling strong. That's good" (period). "So maybe he's getting better!" was not allowed. Or, "Hmm. His breathing sounds more labored tonight, and he's struggling a little more. That's disappointing" (period). Not, "Oh, no, he's getting worse!" I had to gently pull myself back from constant projections of success or doom.

At times I would become sheepishly conscious of my unintentional resemblance to a then-popular but annoying cell-phone commercial: "How are you feeling now? How are you feeling *now*? How about now? *Now*?"

When we combine hypervigilance with overgeneralization, we end up forgetting that we all have normal variances in how we feel. Sometimes I am too achy to ride my bike, and I quit my workout after ten minutes. Sometimes I am out of breath after climbing a flight of stairs. I wouldn't attribute these minor deviations from my usual condition to a deterioration in my health. Therefore it wasn't helpful to either of us when I watched

Bill like a hawk for any clues as to how he was doing at any given moment and, worse yet, treated them as omens for our future.

> Overgeneralization is one of the twelve cognitive distortions de-scribed by Aaron Beck, MD, a psychiatrist who developed cogni-tive behavioral therapy.[18] We are all prone to making certain types of recurring errors in the way we think, and these errors contribute to anxiety and depression. According to the principles of cognitive ther-apy, if we can identify our cognitive distortions and correct them, our thoughts will no longer have the ability to create unwarranted nega-tive emotions. For example, when Laura was able to recognize her tendency to make overgeneralizations, she corrected her thoughts, making them more factual and less emotionally powerful.
>
> There are many self-help books based on the principles of cognitive behavioral therapy. One of my favorites is by David Burns, MD. His self-help book is called *Feeling Good: The New Mood Therapy*,[19] and he also has written *The Feeling Good Handbook*, which takes the reader through a variety of mental exercises in order to practice recognizing and changing dysfunctional thought patterns.[20]

Trusting Yourself

> *Once we believe in ourselves, we can risk*
> *curiosity, wonder, spontaneous delight, or any*
> *experience that reveals the human spirit.*
> —E. E. CUMMINGS

W told me I need to trust in the universe. I may have to work to absorb that idea. But I should certainly be able to have trust in myself. Today I

---

18 Ibid.

19 David D. Burns, *Feeling Good: The New Mood Therapy* (New York: William Morrow and Company, 1980).

20 David D. Burns, *The Feeling Good Handbook*, rev. ed. (New York: Penguin Putnam, 1999).

am 45, a good time to trust that I will handle what comes my way. Trust that I will deal with my future when it comes, without trying to experience it in advance. Trust that I will manage each day as I reach that day. Trust that I can handle my life.

Have faith in your own courage. I found I was much braver than I ever expected I would be. When I saw people in the cancer center with visible symptoms of their illnesses or side effects of their treatment, I would shudder with dread about what it would be like if Bill had similar reactions or setbacks. And when he did, I handled it. Treading unfamiliar waters was very difficult, but I knew it was crucial for me to solidify my conviction that I could handle whatever happened.

One of my concerns as we made tough decisions was whether I would later regret things we chose or didn't choose, longing for the road not taken. At times I would mentally have a conversation with my future self, instructing her not to judge what my current self was doing. Almost as a preemptive strike against future self-doubt or recriminations, I explained to the future me that I was making the best decisions I could, given the information I had at the time. This had worked for me on a couple of earlier occasions in my life when I had been faced with difficult choices that would have huge ramifications on the course of my life.

For example, early in the treatment, we were given a choice. Bill could begin with either chemotherapy or surgery, and like with most medical decisions, there were pros and cons to each of these options. We chose the chemo. Later, when he did have the surgery, we wondered whether we had waited too long to derive the full benefit of that procedure.

I had to mentally stop myself from having remorse about our original choice by reminding myself that we'd made the decision that seemed best at the time given the relative benefits and risks presented to us. I forced myself to keep my own promise that I wouldn't reassess the situation in retrospect. There was nothing to be gained by wondering about the path we hadn't taken. The same was true of all the treatments we chose along the way. We had to weigh the information, which usually wasn't much, without the benefit of data or hindsight. This became a matter of trusting myself: trusting my current self to do my best, trusting my future self not to judge.

It was terrifying and intimidating to be faced with major decisions that might affect the course of Bill's medical condition. Since most of Bill's options were newer treatments or off-label, the doctors refrained from giving us advice, because evidence pointing to a preferred path simply wasn't available. Most of the time, the doctors would lay out the options but then leave the choice to us. I felt that I was playing a giant game of Russian roulette. It was frustrating not to get direction from people who we believed had more information than we did. In today's litigious society, it is understandable that medical personnel may be more reluctant to make specific recommendations without hard evidence. In addition, with so many new treatments constantly being introduced, the data we crave often don't exist. Many times our own family member is providing that data for future patients.

You do the best you can, and that's all you can do. I strongly advise that you promise yourself you will respect and honor the decisions you make. If it appears later that another choice may have been better, be as supportive of yourself as you would be if you were reassuring your best friend if he questioned, down the road, the course he had taken. You know you would be nonjudgmental and comforting to your friend. Be the same way with yourself.

> When I have these thoughts (How would I handle this? How would I handle that?), I have to keep in mind that if you had asked me in January how I would handle Bill getting diagnosed with cancer, it would have been unimaginable. But the reality is that I am handling it, just like I will continue to handle things in my life. If I had started practicing six months or a year ago what I would do if Bill got diagnosed with cancer, it wouldn't have helped me at all in dealing with it now. Months of agonizing wouldn't have made me more adept at managing the reality. I will deal with whatever I need to...I already am.

Mindfulness

I know of no more encouraging fact than
the unquestionable ability of man to
elevate his life by conscious endeavor.
—HENRY DAVID THOREAU

Today I had some success. When I was with Bill and my mind started to
wander, I said to myself, "I choose to be here." It actually worked, helping
me to shed my anxieties and speculation about what is to come.

When our son was seven years old, he had a difficult time falling asleep every night. Bedtime became an arduous and stressful process, sometimes lasting hours, as he repeatedly reemerged from his room despite our various strategies designed to keep him in his bed. Aware of his father's serious illness, he clearly was experiencing anxiety, and while he held everything together by day, he seemed to be engulfed by fears at night.

Many people gave me advice about how to calm and soothe his racing thoughts. A commonly suggested approach was visualizations. Since these types of exercises have never worked for me, it was challenging to try to get my child to focus in this manner. But I tried. When he was in bed, I would make up a scene for him to imagine: "We are on the beach in Mexico. The waves are gently lapping by your feet. Birds are flying overhead. The sun is beginning to go down." I would strain to think up images to get him to concentrate on this idyllic scene to substitute for the tensions in his life that were beyond our control.

It didn't work. I was convinced that I was just bad at evoking visions. But one day I described this failure to a colleague, a psychiatrist who has worked in the area of mindfulness. She told me my mistake was in offering up visualizations that were too expansive. Instead of focusing the mind, they actually provided open, fertile ground for bad thoughts to take hold. In addition, for some people, trying to imagine the perfect scene can be stressful or may bring forth painful memories.

This colleague told me that in order to focus my son's mind in a way that would buffer him from intrusive thoughts, I needed to narrow his concentration rather than expand it. She told me to put something in his room that he could look at for an extended period of time. On the wall next to his bed, I put up a poster of several basketball players. Then we began a nighttime ritual we called "noticing." We took turns commenting on the photo:

"I notice that three of the players are wearing black shoes, and the other four are wearing white."

"I notice that one player has a goatee, one has a mustache, and the rest are clean-shaven."

"I notice that four of the players have tattoos."

This went on for five to ten minutes. After saying good night to my child, I told him to continue noticing until he fell asleep. Every now and then, I moved another poster to this spot.

Most nights our new ritual worked to keep him in bed. Going through this process with my son made me understand how sometimes the best way to be mindful is to reduce the universe into a tiny fragment. By concentrating on one little piece, the jumble of overwhelming thoughts can be cleared to the side. When I am at work and have three or four things going at once, sometimes I have to push everything on my desk to one side or the other so that I can direct my attention to the one thing I have set in the middle to undertake, such as working on a budget or editing a document.

Confronting my husband's illness forced me, like my child, to truly be mindful and to learn to restrict the unfettered access of any random thought into my brain. In order to be a competent gatekeeper, I had to train myself to maximize my focus and concentration.

Grounding techniques can be very helpful in keeping the mind focused. Sit in a chair, and feel your feet solidly on the floor. Touch things with your fingers, and notice the textures. Look around the room, and pay attention to small details: a crack in the paint, the way the breeze makes the curtains flutter, the candy dish that belonged to your grandmother. Listen to sounds: the dull din of the traffic outside, the sound of the fan running in the other room, the chirping bird on the cable line. What are the smells? Stale coffee on the burner, damp grass from last night's rain, and the faint aroma of the cleaning solution just used to wipe down the counter. Ground yourself in the here and now.

Another way to reduce stress is to practice breathing exercises. Put your hand on your stomach, and feel its rise and fall with each breath. Although it may feel awkward at first, try to force your belly to rise with the inhale and fall with the exhale. Slow down the pace, and focus only on this simple process. When upsetting thoughts begin to intrude, bring your mind back to the flow of your breathing. Try this during middle-of-the-night awakenings when your mind is too active to fall back to sleep.

> Mindfulness is a concept derived from meditation. In meditation, mindfulness means maintaining awareness on the breath or on a single image or phrase (a mantra) and returning to that focus every time the mind strays. Mindfulness helps slow and focus the mind, induces a calm state, and can be applied to many situations.

> For example, if you are annoyed that your family went off for the day and left their dirty dishes in the sink, instead of approaching the dishes with resentment, which might provoke you to bang them around, you can choose to turn your mind to the act of washing. Every time your thoughts veer off toward an angry comment about ungrateful family members, you refocus on the warmth of the water, the feel of the sponge against the plate, the pleasing fragrance of the dish soap. Washing the dishes becomes a soothing, sensual experience. When you're done, you may feel calmer, pleased with the good job you've done, and ready to remind your family about good kitchen etiquette with a kind tone of voice when they get home. If that feels unacceptable to you, you could choose to leave the dishes for others to wash, while still

applying mindfulness to your intention not to flare with resentment each time you see the sink full of dishes.

Mindfulness is a way to quiet the mind and permits one to steer toward more pleasing experiences. When responding to upsetting news, a person could choose to do something to calm down. It could be as simple as brewing a cup of tea while staying focused on each little action: filling the kettle with water, turning on the stove, measuring the tea, and so forth. The five minutes it takes to make a cup of tea, when focused mindfully, will serve as a mini respite from anger, worry, grief, or whatever emotion upset you. Now, from this calmer state of mind, the problem can be reevaluated.

Modern life is often hectic, even more so when making room for managing an illness. Multitasking, the opposite of mindfulness, invites a further sense of being harried and fragmented. If mindfulness can be applied to certain activities, the activity becomes a ritual capable of restoring serenity. Folding laundry, feeding the dog, sweeping the floor, and even walking to the mailbox can become opportunities for noticing color, texture, aroma, sounds, your body's movements, and your breathing. Mindfulness turns the chore into a small time-out, an opportunity to feel restored and satisfied.

Living Your Old Life Too

Before enlightenment, chop wood, carry water;
after enlightenment, chop wood, carry water.
—ZEN SAYING

Yesterday Bill and I had a long talk about a drama going on at A's school. It felt like we hadn't processed something so trivial in such a long time. When I mentioned this to E, she said, "I bet a month ago, you thought you would never have a conversation like that again." She was right. It felt nice to get lost in regular life like normal people.

I found that living the new normal and dealing with the new challenges wasn't my only task. I had to live my old life, too.

Life events, big and small, continue to happen. We celebrate holidays and birthdays. We go to recitals, sporting events, school, and work functions. Our children learn to read, start to drive, get married. Other loved ones develop their own health problems. Friends share their joys and sorrows. Everyday life continues. Every day, life continues.

I remember listening to a radio commentary by Kenneth Turan, film critic for the *Los Angeles Times*, after 9-11 on the question of whether it was frivolous for people to go to the movies in the aftermath of such a tragic event. He talked about having gone to Sarajevo years earlier and being surprised at how invested people were in going to movies even during the siege of the city. Seeing films gave the citizens the simple thing they had been most denied: the sense of being normal.

The first Sarajevo film festival took place during the siege, and the organizer was asked by journalists, "Why a film festival during the war?"

He responded, "Why a war during the film festival?"

I thought about this story when I wanted to keep perspective about the normal part of our lives. Our older daughter turned sixteen on the day of Bill's first treatment.

"Why a fondue party on the first day of chemo?"

"Why chemo on the day of our fondue party?"

> *The sad part about today was listening to everyone talk about their up-coming vacations. The hard thing about trying to live in the moment is that, in reality, you want to feel like everyone else. "We, too, are planning our trip" (god willing, god willing, god willing). We need to balance the desire and necessity to be in the present with the desire and necessity to be normal, think ahead, and plan.*

Bill and I were committed to not letting his cancer take away everything that was ordinary in our lives. In fact, on the day we had our first meeting with the oncologist, we dragged ourselves home, scared and exhausted. Bill insisted I go to my book-group meeting that night. Wanting to be home with him and the kids, I resisted. "You have to do it for me," he pleaded. "I need to see you do normal things."

Another time, shortly after his diagnosis, I was discussing with an acquaintance our plans for our younger daughter's bat mitzvah, which was a year away. She asked me how I could even think about that right now. I remember feeling stubborn in answering, "How can I not?" We needed to still be us, to feel the promise of the future.

Even though there were times we had to change our priorities to deal with new developments, it was important for us not to step entirely out of the structure of what was routine, familiar, and necessary.

> The idea of making the illness adapt to your life rather than adapting your life to the illness may seem strange, even delusional, but it is actually very sensible. The familiar, old routines and social events provide the basic rhythm or structure of our daily, weekly, and seasonal lives. It is around the scaffolding of the same routines and rituals that one constructs the new life of the patient or caregiver.

> While some events and commitments may need to be changed or set aside, it is comforting to retain the same basic rhythm in daily life. The process of evaluating what to keep, what to modify, and what to discard can be exhilarating. You finally have an excuse to step down from the committee you don't enjoy, but you'll hold on to your monthly book club, because it's fun. Dropping all your regular routines and activities would leave you without the pacing and support to which you have been accustomed, and now is the time when you most need that support.

When we care for loved ones, another intrusion on our normal lifestyle is when we allow equipment and medications to take over our homes. To the extent that it is at all feasible, try to put away the accoutrements that are constant reminders of the illness or disability. It is depressing to continually look at a row of pill bottles lined up along the kitchen counter or a bedpan on the nightstand. Obviously you can't remove everything from view, but the more you can, the more you can maintain some semblance of normality. The sights and smells of a sick house can intimidate visitors and strip your loved one of his or her dignity. Eliminating or reducing offensive odors as much as possible is especially important. Our environments affect our moods. While tidiness is usually not our most pressing concern, the psychological effect of the clutter of illness can be an emotional noose.

CHAPTER 4

Managing Emotional Responses

Y ou may be experiencing many emotions, and their intensity may be difficult at times. In this chapter, we discuss the range of emotions people encounter when dealing with a loved one's illness. Don't worry about whether your emotions are "normal"; they are your experience, and they are real. We offer suggestions for how to allow yourself to feel what you're feeling, and we describe adaptive ways to manage those feelings.

Anxiety

> *I am not afraid of storms, for I am*
> *learning how to sail my ship.*
> —Louisa May Alcott

When anxiety grabs us, it can be a full sweep of mind and body. The symptoms are often so visceral that many people end up in emergency rooms, as they mistake anxiety for a serious physical illness, such as a heart attack. The tightening of the chest, the quick pulsing of the heart, and the abdominal pain of anxiety can easily mimic other illnesses. The bodily sensations might be so tangible that a psychological cause doesn't even occur to the person who is feeling them.

There is an interesting paradox to anxiety. At times the phenomenon can cause us to be completely out of touch with the emotions that may dwell beneath the surface of our physical sensations. In other instances, it forcefully jars us into an awareness of how connected our emotional and physical worlds are.

Anxiety can be all-consuming and relentless. When our minds race and ruminate, we find that we are projecting unproductively and obsessively into the future, a future over which we have very little control. When we become preoccupied with rehearsing our future responses or regretting past events, we rob ourselves of our current experience, which is, in fact, all we really have. With the past and the future both vying for prominent positions in our psyches, what happens to the present? If it is suppressed into insignificance, how can we be surprised when we find we are disconnected from our own existence? And furthermore, how can we not feel even more anxious when we become aware of this self-estrangement?

A troubling and often debilitating outcome of obsessive thinking is sleeplessness. Many caregivers experience the inability to calm the racing mind and employ strategies from breathing exercises to sleeping pills in order to block anxiety from preventing sleep. For sufferers of insomnia, the impact can be far ranging, from fatigue to irritability to underperformance to disordered thinking. Quality of life becomes collateral damage.

One common form of obsessive thinking is catastrophizing. We work ourselves into a frenzy, in which we imagine all that can go wrong and thus compound our thoughts into an uncontrollable disaster. If we are lucky, we can sometimes take this tactic to an extreme that ultimately stops the madness. This can happen when we project every possible bad outcome to a level of awareness where we can actually see the fallacy of our assumptions and conclusions. Perhaps by hitting bottom with our thoughts, we can actually connect to that ground. We recover our senses and reclaim our experiences.

In the last chapter, I discussed the strategy of compartmentalization. For some people, this strategy works well to contain worry.

For others, it is ineffective. Some people are soothed by a paradoxical process called "flooding." They allow their thoughts to travel quickly down the cascade of worst-case scenarios until they get to the very end. The terminus of the worst-case scenario is often absurd, and recognizing this absurdity relieves anxiety.

For example, a woman who is the primary caregiver for her ill mother may feel overcome by worry that she'll be immobilized by grief if her mother dies. If encouraged to imagine that immobilization to the worst possible outcome, she may envision being unable to get out of bed, in which case she won't be able to feed her children, and then the whole family will starve to death.

At this point, she is likely to realize that while she may in fact not get out of bed for a day or two, friends or other family will feed the children, and nobody will starve to death. Furthermore, if she really can't get out of bed after a few days, other people will intervene, perhaps by taking her to the doctor.

Flooding is a very effective technique for addressing anxiety, but it should never be forced on anyone. When a therapist uses the flooding technique, it is after educating the patient about the process and obtaining the patient's consent. This technique is not comfortable for everyone; for some people, it may be just too overwhelming.

Grief

> *Give sorrow words: the grief that does not speak*
> *Whispers the o'er fraught heart, and bids it break.*
> —WILLIAM SHAKESPEARE, *MACBETH*

Tonight I went to a lecture by Anne Lamott. She spoke quite a bit about grief and losing people you love. I started to tear up as though I recognized these feelings of grief. But then I felt like an imposter. These feelings didn't belong to me; my loved one is very much alive. Why was I tearing up? Because I might lose him? Well, that was always the case. I was tearing up because I now have to think about these things. I, a month ago, would have heard her stories of grief in a detached way: it's interesting but doesn't apply to me. Now it seems like everything sad applies.

In the course of her talk, Anne said, "There's more room in a broken heart." This resonated with me, because that is how I feel. My heart is broken, because I no longer have the confidence in what kind of future I have with Bill. My heart is broken as I overhear people planning graduations and weddings, talking about grandchildren, anything that involves happy moments in the future, which holds such uncertainty for me. The "more room" speaks to me because I do sense an exit of so many petty annoyances, minor obsessions, and worries, leaving more space for the things that matter.

I found that it was important not to reject my feelings, even when they were uncomfortably or painfully intense. Letting myself feel my grief was fundamental to working through it and getting to a place of acceptance and healing. After Bill was diagnosed with cancer, it took me a while to realize that the weighty sadness I was feeling was actually grief. While my instincts were to push those difficult emotions aside and stay focused, I came to understand that it wasn't helpful to completely shun my natural and justifiable sadness.

"Feel your feelings" was a gentle refrain from my therapist. Sometimes I found myself repeating those words in my head to move past the barrier of my defenses and let the emotional impact of what I was experiencing flow through my consciousness.

It is a common misconception that people feel grief only after a death. In fact, grief occurs after many kinds of losses, including loss of a job, a home, a limb, or health. Grief is a heavy, sad feeling; it may be accompanied by tightness or heaviness in one's chest, which may be the origin of the phrase "a broken heart." It is an extreme version of sadness or sorrow.

Sometimes grief is hard to distinguish from depression, a clinical condition in which a person is relentlessly sad, often with physical manifestations, such as inability to sleep through the night, poor appetite, low concentration, low energy, and increased physical pain. A person with depression may have diminished self-esteem, inappropriate and excessive guilt, and suicidal thoughts, which are usually not elements of grief. Grief, which is a natural condition, may metamorphose into major depression, which is a medical condition that requires treatment.

A lot has been written about grief, most famously in the book *On Death and Dying: What the Dying Have to Teach Doctors, Nurses, Clergy and Their Own Families*, by Elisabeth Kübler-Ross, a Swiss-born psychiatrist who practiced in the United States.[21] Some authors imply that one must grieve "correctly" or suffer consequences down the road. The way one grieves is as unique as the way one loves, differing according to one's personality, the nature of the loss, the timing of the loss, and other factors. One's grief is likely to feel different and be expressed differently depending on whether the loss was abrupt or anticipated; whether it was a solitary loss, the third loss in six months, or an ongoing loss, such as the gradual diminishing of ability in a person with a degenerative disease; and whether the person had earlier losses that were not resolved.

Will this life ever feel normal again? I feel like there is a constant throbbing that never totally subsides. People learn to live with constant physical pain or discomfort. Do you just learn to live with the emotional equivalent of that, too?

I couldn't always predict what might make me sad. Sometimes the occasions I most dreaded, like a holiday or birthday celebrated with Bill in a weakened condition, ended up being more manageable than I anticipated.

---

21   Elisabeth Kübler-Ross, *On Death and Dying: What the Dying Have to Teach Doctors, Nurses, Clergy and Their Own Families* (New York: Macmillan, 1969).

Meanwhile, an everyday nonevent might send me into an emotional tail-spin. The first time we went to the mountains after Bill's diagnosis, I prepared myself that he likely wouldn't have the stamina for a hike, but I didn't foresee that he would struggle with the stairs to the walkway over the highway. I was ready for the sadness I felt attending a family event while he was home resting after chemo, but I didn't expect the sadness I felt one morning watching our son's soccer game by myself while Bill slept in. I had to learn to accept that sometimes my sad feelings would be unpredictable and unexpected. And I had to have the courage to let myself feel them.

> *Yesterday I pep talked myself out of experiencing a sad moment and tried to convince myself to find the joy in the situation. But really I think I just needed to feel sad. This is my dilemma. How much and how often do I let myself feel sad, and when do I cut it off? When do I try to lift myself up, and when do I allow myself to sink? How do I strike that balance?*

> *Today our new dining-room table finally came, 12 weeks after I ordered it. I just felt numb and even ambivalent about it. I am no longer the same person who ordered that table. Three months ago, I ran all over town looking at and measuring dozens of tables. But now that it is here, I feel nothing, like its whole purchase was frivolous and meaningless. And I am sad, because it represents a me I don't feel like anymore, a me who so enthusiastically bought the table and was thrilled upon finding the perfect chairs on clearance at another store.*

> *I know I shouldn't try to talk myself out of the sadness by arguing that I wouldn't want to be that person whose biggest excitement was a new table. But I would want to be her again. I do want to be the person who could take delight in projecting years and years of bringing friends and family around my dinner table. I want to be the untroubled person I was 12 weeks ago.*

Naming Your Loss

There is no pain so great as the
memory of joy in present grief.
—AESCHYLUS

When Bill was first diagnosed, I found myself grieving. But at the same time, I didn't know exactly what to grieve, since Bill was alive and doing well. I started to grieve the loss of him and our relationship even when I was sitting right next to him. Then I would kick myself for prematurely conducting a process that might not be necessary for many years to come. It felt wrong and even unseemly to have these thoughts. I would reprimand myself for wasting our precious time together. Yet I was dealing with grief and couldn't figure out how to appropriately handle it. Gradually, I learned to acknowledge and work through my grief and to really name exactly what it was. Although it was inappropriate to grieve the loss of Bill, I could grieve other things.

For example, a friend told me she was planning a sailing trip with her husband "not this summer but next summer." I grieved that I wasn't able to plan a trip with my husband two years away. Another friend told me she was sorry she hadn't responded to a call, but she was dealing with a work crisis and would be "back to normal next week." I grieved that I wouldn't be back to normal next week. A colleague described in detail a house she and her husband were building in New Hampshire so that they could "retire in five years." I grieved that I couldn't even imagine what my life would be like in five years. A friend delighted in the birth of his first grandchild. I grieved Bill's low odds of seeing one of our children get married, let alone the arrival of a grandchild.

What I am feeling is a loss of innocence. My carefree life has been cut off and replaced by a realization that my dreams and expectations are in deep jeopardy. I also grieve a loss of innocence for the kids. No matter the outcome, they will endure the weight and sadness of their father's illness, an experience we hoped they wouldn't have to face for decades. I grieve the loss of my assumptions. I grieve that there is so much I can't share with Bill when I am used to sharing everything with him. I grieve that I have to spend so much time writing in this journal because I don't want to burden him with my sadness. I grieve that I have this sadness. I grieve that my calendar is full of appointments saying "chemo" and "CT scan."

I guess it comes down to grieving that we are dealing with this. Our life feels so vulnerable—this is what I grieve.

It wasn't necessary to open Pandora's box and grieve every piece of my life that I could possibly lose. But when something came up that felt like a potential loss, I gave myself permission to experience the grief.

With focus and effort, I learned how to name my grief very specifically. Precise grieving allows you to experience *real* losses without mourning those that may or may not occur. You may grieve the loss of your expectations for the future, the loss of your loved one's health, the impact this situation is having on your children, parents, or friends. You might feel the loss of your optimism, your hopes and dreams, and your sense of security.

And working through some of these feelings of grief as they occur may ultimately be helpful if, God forbid, the worst-case scenario comes to pass. Although it is not something you want or need to think about now, grief work done today can give you a head start if you end up needing to grieve the ultimate loss. This type of grieving is different from the unproductive worrying mentioned in previous chapters. Here you allow yourself to experience real losses occurring in your life.

In the case of a particularly bad prognosis, there may be times when you can't help but jump ahead a bit and allow yourself to dip your toes in and test the waters of what it might feel like if you were grieving your loved one's death. This anticipatory grief gives your psyche a chance to anticipate the loss, as opposed to the shock it suffers when it is thrown into the depths of grief in the case of a sudden, unexpected loss.

Anticipatory grief is not the same as giving up. As you adapt to your loved one's illness, you may at times find yourself imagining life without him or her. A wave of sadness or loneliness or even relief may wash over you. This is anticipatory grief, and it is a natural process of adaptation. Human intelligence permits us to imagine and plan for the future. In this way, we scout out the path ahead of us and prepare for what might lie ahead.

A woman who takes care of her son who is a quadriplegic after a spinal-cord injury may find herself daydreaming about how life will be different after her son is no longer here. She'll have time to see friends again, go on vacations, and pursue old hobbies. Her fantasies and plans for the future don't mean she wants her son to die, but they are her way of anticipating and consoling herself about how hard it is to watch her son's incapacity. If her son dies or moves to a long-term-care facility, she will have already visited in her mind the feelings of grief and loneliness, and she will also have mapped out some ideas about how to cope and what to do next.

Inviting the Sadness

> *Into each life some rain must fall,*
> *Some days must be dark and dreary.*
> —HENRY WADSWORTH LONGFELLOW

I know that grief is a process, but how long do I need to be sad for this process to start working? How many hours a day? How many months? Bill asks me to enjoy the time we have together, and he is right. But I have so many things to balance: to feel my sadness but not show it very much; to feel my sadness but not every single second; to feel my sadness but (and?) appreciate our good times and make the most of them.

Sometimes I felt pent-up grief and couldn't figure out how to release it. I wanted to feel my own pain, but I needed help getting it out of the deep place where I tended to subconsciously stuff it. In my effort to hold things together, I often felt that I was out of touch with the part of me that was terribly sad. This would make me feel inauthentic and even guilty. When I was able to pull it out of myself, I felt better in the same way you feel better after you throw up. It can be wrenching going through the process, but that wasted feeling you have when it is over actually can be cathartic and calming. And when I refer to the "process," sometimes it was only a few minutes. It didn't have to be a whole morning or day of suffering. Just enough to get that needed relief.

But how did I pull it out? I found a couple of sad songs that, when I put them on, would always make me cry. I would write in my journal and discover my own grief as the words flew across the page. I would look at pictures of happy times before we lived in the shadow of the illness.

It can feel like a dichotomy to pursue two seemingly inconsistent purposes at the same time. On the one hand, I wanted to be positive and manage gracefully. On the other, I wanted to access my grief so that I could experience it and work through it. There were times when I wondered if, in my effort to mirror Bill's optimism, I was suppressing my own grief. What a tricky balancing act! Somehow I was able to convince myself that I could be both hopeful and sad, just maybe not at the exact same moment.

We are so accustomed to pushing away unpleasant thoughts or experiences. It feels counterintuitive to intentionally bring on something we know will be painful. But getting in touch with those feelings that inevitably dwell within us can help to deflate the impact they have on our psyches, however subtle.

When I write in this journal, I force myself to evoke my emotions and feel my feelings. Like a difficult workout, the goal is that I will end up in a healthier place. But it is not like I purge these feelings and they're gone. They fill right back up, like the fluid in Bill's lung.

Sometimes people are afraid that if they start to cry, they won't be able to stop. This is an irrational fear. It is important to create a safe place for grief, to allow yourself enough time to feel your feelings, cry, and recover before the next scheduled life task. It may help to create a ritual that opens and closes a grieving session. For example, park your car by the side of the road and put on a favorite song that elicits your feelings to begin your grieving. Then change to another song that elicits hope or courage, reapply your lipstick (if you wear it) or straighten your tie (if you wear one), and drive to your next destination. Perhaps you want to stop by a grocery store for an apple with which to nourish yourself?

The Kübler-Ross Stages

One may not reach the dawn save by the path of the night.
—Kahlil Gibran

In discussions with people and in your readings, you will likely come across the five stages of grief. In some less sophisticated articles or summaries, they are presented as almost a recipe you must follow in order to reach the desired outcome of healthy adjustment. Although it was helpful for me to understand the range of normal feelings people experience, I also learned that everyone is different.

Sometimes, when I read books that would detail the way I was supposed to feel, I actually needed reassurance if I didn't appear to fit the usual patterns. I worried that I wasn't reacting or responding right or in the right order or to the right degree and that a failure to undergo the different phases or stages correctly could screw me up in the future. When it came to grieving, I was my usual overachieving self, eager to do what I was supposed to do in order to be successful at my task. But when my emotions didn't neatly fit the prescribed path, I found the support I needed to recognize that my own instincts were just fine.

Grief has many outward manifestations. Elisabeth Kübler-Ross described five stages of grief that she had observed in her patients: denial, bargaining, anger, depression, and acceptance.[22] She later clarified that people do not necessarily go through these stages in a linear fashion; rather, people visit some or all of the stages in any order and may revisit a stage they have already experienced. The stages of grief may be triggered by one's own illness or approaching death, the death or illness of a loved one, divorce, or any other loss. Each of the five elements of grief is briefly described in this section.

Denial

As discussed in chapter 2, denial may be the initial reaction we have to adversity. It is the response of "This is not really happening," which serves as an initial buffer to the shock and upset of bad news. Usually this stage is worked through fairly rapidly, often by moving to the stage of bargaining. When a person stays in denial and cannot progress to another stage of grief, problems in adaptation may arise.

Maintaining a modicum of denial, if needed, to fuel your hopefulness is not a problem, as long as denial is not the only response you employ.

Bargaining

The transition from denial to bargaining is simple. It is easy to go from "This isn't happening" to "I promise to go to church every Sunday if this goes away" or "Please let my loved one live to see my child graduate from high school." People offer a pact with God or the universe or fate or whatever power they identify, essentially offering to accept the loss they are facing if they can name the terms. Bargaining is an attempt to regain a measure of control at a time when the person feels he or she has lost control.

---

22 Ibid.

Anger

Our culture tends to view anger as something bad or harmful, something to be avoided. Yet anger is a natural response to loss, and it has adaptive qualities. In grief, anger may sound like "Why me? This isn't right!" It can lend energy to the fighting spirit that seems so beneficial to people when faced with hardship.

If a person is unable to work through his or her anger, to turn it in an adaptive direction, it may interfere with the ability to respond effectively to the situation at hand. When a medically ill person directs his or her anger at a treatment provider, for example, it may interfere with the ability to communicate and collaborate concerning medical care. If the spouse of an ailing person directs his or her anger about the illness at the person facing the illness, both people will be miserable.

Sometimes it is more comfortable for a person to feel anger than sadness. Anger is associated with energy, and it is usually expressed outward, as opposed to the inward-turning and depleting experience of sadness. For many people, it is easier to separate from someone in anger than in sadness. We see this often in adolescence, when the teenager departs for summer camp or college in a storm of rage to avoid feeling sad about leaving the familiarity and comfort of the parental home. If a person is very uncomfortable experiencing sadness, then the grieving process may get stuck in anger.

Depression

Kübler-Ross describes the depression stage of grief as hopelessness: "Why bother trying? What's the point?" This is not the same as the clinical diagnosis of major depression, which requires treatment and which we discuss in chapter 7. Depression as a stage of grief involves sadness and despair, but it generally does not include other symptoms of major depression, such as poor concentration, diminished self-esteem, excessive guilt, lack of capacity to experience pleasure, or suicidal thoughts. With support, a person in the depressed stage of grief can usually find the answer to "Why bother trying?" and move forward toward acceptance and healthy adaptation.

It is common for people to cycle back and forth between the depressed stage and the angry stage, oscillating between outrage and despair in response to ongoing developments in the challenges they face. It is also possible to come back to anger or despair even after having achieved Kübler-Ross's final stage: acceptance.

Acceptance

When you are able to acknowledge the loss or crisis in a way that helps you deal with it, you have arrived at acceptance: "This is a problem that won't go away by itself, so I'm going to address it." Acceptance is very different from giving up. Giving up belongs to the stage of depression. Acceptance permits one to develop a realistic plan or strategy for addressing the crisis.

Other Emotional Challenges

I will love the light for it shows me the way, yet I will endure the darkness for it shows me the stars.
—OG MANDINO

In addition to the emotions we have already discussed, such as sadness and anger, we often find our mood dipping into other territories, sometimes familiar, sometimes unexpected. This section does not cover all the potential mood changes we may encounter but addresses some of the ones that are commonly experienced while supporting a loved one who is ill.

Mood Variances

I have been feeling more on edge. I know I am driving the whole family crazy with my hypervigilance. I have to figure out a way to keep myself from constantly boarding this emotional roller coaster and riding Bill's condition of the moment. Yesterday I was upbeat when he came back from the gym reporting a run in which he felt better than he has in a long time. Then I plummeted last night when he was gasping while talking, coughing, and breathing hard and shallow. I keep watching him like a vulture, making every change a sign of our future. This is going to be a sure way to drive all of us crazy.

I found my mood to be a moving target, closely following Bill's condition. When he felt good and thought his treatment was working, I would feel light and cheerful. When he had trouble breathing and felt like he was getting worse, I would get distressed and anxious.

Outwardly, I rarely revealed the inner turmoil I was experiencing. These wide mood variances I was feeling were uncomfortable and exhausting. Hopeful, fearful, sad, content: this psychological flitting around required a great deal of energy. Since I have always thought of myself as having an even-keeled temperament, the internal highs and lows I was experiencing felt foreign, and it became necessary for me to absorb these deviations into my reality. I also found myself grappling with other unpleasant emotions, such as fear and guilt.

Fear

I recognized the pit I felt in my stomach as fear. I was afraid of what was going to happen in my life. I remembered a family vacation where we'd walked across one of those wobbly suspension bridges right over a gorge. Out in the middle of the bridge, I felt a panic, a momentary paralysis. But of course there was no choice except to continue across.

When we find ourselves exposed like this in life, we may be unnerved by fear, but there is no turning back; we must keep moving. When anxiety about the unknown becomes overwhelming, we have to remind ourselves that we *never have known* what the future would bring. Dealing with illness can be very threatening, pulling us abruptly and completely out of our comfort zones. When we tread the narrow bridges in our lives, we need to keep in mind that we can go only forward, one step at a time.

Fear can certainly become debilitating, but sometimes it can have a galvanizing influence. When you read in the news about people who commit heroic acts, they often describe an adrenalin-induced surge that provides the motivation and ability to behave in a way they never thought possible. Mental-health experts often talk about the fight, flight, and freeze aspects of fear. When the fight mechanism is activated, fear can bring out your innate survival instincts. Find the ways to harness your fear and turn it into a source of strength and drive. Keep in mind, of course, that this hyperalert state is not a healthy place to stay. If you are unable to move from that jittery, aroused frame of mind, it is time to do some grounding exercises, talk to a friend, or seek help from a therapist.

Frustration

Many people who find themselves in caregiving roles find irritability an unwelcome companion on the journey. A man I knew took care of his wife, who had neuropathy in her hands as one of many symptoms of her illness. This condition caused her to drop things and also limited her ability to pick up the resulting messes effectively. He described an occasion in which she dropped a jar of beads that broke all over the kitchen floor. The husband lashed out at her as he began separating the glass shards from the beads she wanted salvaged.

In relating the story to me, he acknowledged sincere remorse for yelling at his wife, who had intended no harm, but he felt he was "at wit's end" with having his own activities being continuously interrupted by her clumsiness. He knew it was unfair to fault her, but his aggravation was human and honest, especially given the frequency of these occasions. Ultimately, telling the story to an empathic listener allowed him to unload some of his stress, bolstering him to reengage with his spouse with compassion. Again, these are times to find effective coping strategies and resources to ward off resentment and discover alternative ways to respond to times when we become understandably frustrated.

Distraction

In the early days and weeks of adjusting to the news of the diagnosis, I had a hard time concentrating on my daily tasks. I became forgetful and would jump from one task to another with little ability to focus. Although I am typically a fairly organized person, I would get late notices for bills I thought I had paid and reminders for school forms I was sure I had turned in. Piles built up on my desk; birthday invitations were neglected. I also found I had memory problems. Did I ask the teacher about a deadline? And if I did, what was the answer?

Many times I felt like it was all I could do to keep handling the bare minimum. It was not a period in my life in which I would have been successful in any new challenges, professionally or personally. When my mind would wander days, weeks, and years beyond the present, I would have to force myself to focus on the task at hand, in the now.

Guilt

There are many reasons we may feel guilt during the time we are supporting a loved one with an illness. It may be as simple as feeling guilty that the person you love is weak or in pain while you are feeling fine and able. Guilt may also arise if you experience anger or resentment toward that person or about the disruption the illness is causing in your lives, leaving you feeling ashamed that you have such emotions about someone who is sick. If your loved one is very demanding, you may feel guilty about the breaks you must take for some respite. When treatment or caregiving becomes expensive, you may feel guilty about worrying about the resources that are being expended. You may feel guilty if you are involved with admitting your loved one to a psychiatric hospital, residential treatment facility, or nursing home. Recognize and validate these emotions, and find ways to work through these feelings so they don't weigh you down. Remind yourself of all the things you are doing to help and care for your loved one. Spare yourself the guilt—it would be unusual if you never had any negative thoughts.

Ambivalence

A common cause of guilt is when caregivers have ambivalent feelings about the outcome of the situation or even about the loved one as a person. There are many reasons why you might feel ambivalent.

The most obvious example is when your loved one is suffering and is not going to get better. You might experience very mixed feelings. On the one hand, you want it to be over and the pain to stop; on the other hand, you aren't ready to let go, and the thought of losing this person is too painful. These are common and often unspoken co-occurring sentiments. Maybe when another heart attack or stroke or setback occurs, you think, *This could be the one*, and you're not sure what you hope will happen.

Even when your loved one is not overtly suffering, you may feel simultaneous conflicting emotions. A friend once told me about caring for her mother with advanced dementia. Once a vibrant woman with loving connections to her children and grandchildren, she now had no recognition of the people who had once been her whole world. Moreover, she could not perform even the most basic skills of self-care, a heartbreaking turn of events for a woman who had always valued her independence. My friend spent countless hours organizing the care of her mother while juggling her own family and her job. And yet her feelings of wanting it all to come to a peaceful end were countered by her enduring attachment. She said, "Sometimes I honestly want her to just pass away peacefully in her sleep. But other times I feel so happy that at least I can still sit with her and hold her hand."

We discuss in chapter 7 the challenges of caregiving when a relationship is difficult or strained. Those are also situations when you may feel ambivalence, this time about the person. Sometimes the best you can do is accept that you have ambivalent feelings and just decide to be OK with that. But if those feelings are interfering with your ability to function in the role you are assuming, you may need to get professional help to work through that conflict.

Displacement

Anybody can become angry—that is easy. But
to be angry with the right person, to the right
degree, at the right time, for the right purpose,
and in the right way—that is not easy.
—ARISTOTLE

When we feel engulfed by the challenges and exhaustion caused by the details we need to track and attend to, it is not uncommon for us to transfer our frustration to a situation or person unrelated to the source of our anxiety or irritation. We start kicking the proverbial dog. We may sit bravely and stoically when the doctor gives us bad news but then burst into tears later at the slightest provocation, such as spilling a cup of coffee or receiving a critical comment from a coworker. Sometimes we are immediately aware of our overreaction; other times, it just snowballs into a feeling that we are walking around with a huge, dark cloud following our every step.

It is important to recognize these moments and realign your perspective. You may need to offer apologies to anyone who may have been the recipient of an unjustified outburst. Most people will understand if you explain why you may have been oversensitive or behaved uncharacteristically.

Taking care of your loved one often entails making sacrifices. You may have to cancel a vacation that you had carefully planned before the illness emerged or take on extra responsibilities you don't like. Your leisure time is likely to be curtailed. These sacrifices may be necessary and appropriate, but they may also make you feel bad.

It is natural to feel angry some of the time. Anger can be used in a productive way if you understand that it is a signal that something feels hard or frustrating and then set about adjusting the situation. For example, when the spouse who ordinarily pays the bills gets sick, the bills may get paid late. If the other spouse responds with anger, that doesn't help the bills get paid in a more timely fashion, but it does signal to the couple that the bill-paying arrangement may need to be renegotiated. If the angry spouse recognizes that the anger is born from anxiety about future financial security because of the illness, then he or she can shift from a position of blame to one of problem-solving: What do we need to do to ensure our financial security in the near and long term?

Sometimes the anger is harder to understand or contain. A man who recently learned he had HIV infection became enraged with his landlord for not responding quickly enough to his call about a broken fixture in his apartment building. The force of his anger interfered with his sleep, and he considered withholding his rent payment in protest. This response was disproportionate and potentially self-destructive, but it took a few sessions of therapy to help the man realize he was actually angry about the diagnosis of HIV. He had been too frightened initially to consider this as the source of his rage.

While this example may seem extreme, it illustrates a common psychological defense to overwhelming or unacceptable emotions: displacement. Displacement is the process by which an emotion, usually anger, is evoked by one person or situation but expressed to another person or situation, because the consequences of expressing it directly are perceived to be too great.

For example, if your boss elicits hostile feelings, you may unconsciously repress those feelings while at work so that you don't lose your job and then permit them to come to the surface when you drive home, yelling at a driver who failed to signal a turn or harshly scolding your son for leaving his bicycle helmet in the front yard. In the example above, the man was really angry with himself for placing himself at risk for HIV infection, but he couldn't initially tolerate feeling this self-directed anger, because he already felt terribly threatened and overwhelmed by the HIV diagnosis. If you find yourself having a disproportionately strong response to a relatively small provocation, consider whether your response is a displacement of feelings that belong to larger concerns that want your attention.

Exposing Your Emotions

Without wearing any mask we are conscious
of, we have a special face for each friend.
—OLIVER WENDELL HOLMES, SR.

Sometimes it is just inconvenient to feel my feelings. I have to learn to compartmentalize so that my sadness doesn't run my life. If I feel a wave at an inopportune time, I can try to mentally stick it away and then summon it up and address it when I have some time and privacy.

Because of Bill's sensitivity and alertness to my emotions, I felt I had to limit how much of my grief I exposed to him. He tended to interpret my sadness as a lack of confidence in his chances of getting better. My anxiety seemed to cause him more anxiety than even his own, so I tried to shield him from most of it by writing in my journal, processing with other people, or just crying in the bathroom.

For the most part, I felt pretty guarded about my sadness and often felt that I had to modulate my response to protect others. At the same time, I knew it was important for me to take care of my own needs and not repress my feelings.

Do you have a person or people to whom you can expose your darkest side? It is helpful for even the most private types to have someone who will listen without judgment, who knows what you need, and who will be comfortable with your expressions of fear or grief.

When you find yourself stammering to answer a simple inquiry as to how you are, remember that you are under no obligation to tell everyone your deepest feelings. Come up with a standard answer if that is easier. Sometimes I too readily shared my innermost feelings with more casual acquaintances and then found myself regretting that I had done so. I began discriminating between the folks with whom I felt safe and comfortable expressing my intimate thoughts and those with whom it felt more appropriate to deliver more of a rehearsed or stock response.

In doing so, I felt that I was being more respectful of our family's privacy than when I found myself revealing descriptive details to everyone who asked. This also cut down on the risk of being pulled into long or difficult conversations that often were not helpful to me and reduced the chance that I would inadvertently put another person in the position of holding an awkward space that he or she might not welcome.

It can be useful to have a standard answer or two that can be efficiently delivered and is honest enough, such as "We're hanging in there," "We're doing pretty well," or "We're holding strong."

And then if you do not want to further engage, try to deflect the focus of the conversation: "And how are you doing?" "And how was your trip?" "So what's happening with your new job?"

Given that my children were young during Bill's illness, I am often asked about the delicate task of keeping them informed while protecting their well-being. For me, it was my instinct to temper how much I allowed them to see. I was aware that they were extremely vigilant about how I was doing and that they might interpret my vulnerability as an inability to ultimately take care of them. I wanted them to feel secure that they would be all right no matter what happened. And it was clear to me that their sense of security was closely related to how they perceived me. If I was OK, they would be OK.

At the same time, I thought it was important for my kids to see some of my grief. A wise friend told me the best thing I could do for my kids was to be real. Knowing that we all have our own emotional makeup and expressive styles, which may change in different circumstances, I was aware that in my various reactions to bad or good news, I was modeling for my children that a wide range of responses can be normal and acceptable. I certainly did not want them to think that there was one correct way for them to behave in times of stress in their lives.

Another thing to keep in mind about kids is that even when you think you know your children very well, they may have thoughts and misconceptions that wouldn't even occur to you. Shortly after Bill's diagnosis, I was reading a booklet that advised parents to reassure children that cancer isn't contagious. It never dawned on me to have this conversation, but I'll never forget the relief on our six-year-old's face when I explained that he could not *catch* cancer from Daddy. I felt terrible that he had apparently been silently carrying this fear with him, unbeknown to all the adults in his life who were desperately trying to protect him from the real fears we were all contemplating.

Strengthening Where You Are Weak

You gain strength, courage, and confidence by every experience in which you really stop to look fear in the face. You must do the thing which you think you cannot do.
—Eleanor Roosevelt

We all tend to have our own natural ways of reacting to stress. We may be wired to go immediately to fear or to anger or to denial or to something else. When we are disoriented, we do what is familiar, even if it doesn't necessarily work well or isn't in our best interests. This is a time when, out of necessity, we may have to confront and manage emotions that are only adding to our distress.

Many of us work out regularly to train our bodies to become stronger, to gear up for physical challenges, and to feel that we are in shape. We are all familiar with the routines we employ to gain control over our physical condition by going to the gym or engaging a personal trainer. When we are under stress, perhaps we need to do the same thing mentally by training our minds to be fit and prepared for emotional challenges.

With equal determination, we can try to master our emotional condition by fortifying the places where we are weak. It takes time and practice, but with intention and purpose, we can enhance our inner being by becoming conscious of negative thought patterns and behaviors that impair our ability to handle the challenges we are facing. By building emotional stamina, we can learn to rely on it. We train ourselves emotionally to face what we need to face.

> *So today a repairman tore apart our laundry room looking for the cause of our huge flood this morning. Just when everything feels as horrible as possible, it gets even worse. As I moved all the junk out of the laundry room and cleaned up all the water, Bill stood helplessly watching—at my insistence, since I didn't want him to exert himself this way. I didn't know whether to feel sorrier for him or for me. Then I spent the better part of the afternoon on a crazy run around town, trying to get some records for his appointment tomorrow. I felt like I wanted to drive off a cliff. I was talking to M today, and she said, "You just have to handle it because you have to." I guess that simple statement says it all. You handle it because you have to—it's not a choice.*

When you have managed to handle something even after you were sure you had hit the wall, it becomes part of you, part of your history. Build on that experience: "I've done it before; I can do it again." I remember early in my college career, I had a paper due that I was absolutely 100 percent sure I would not be able to turn in on time. But like many of my peers, I found myself staying up all night, drinking a lot of coffee, and ultimately turning in a good product. When the scenario repeated itself, I knew that if I had to stay up all night and get an assignment finished, I could, because I had done it before. That assumption was based on experience and proof.

Recent research into the effects of acute and chronic stress show that acute stress can help the individual respond quickly and effectively, by speeding up the heart rate, pumping more oxygen to muscles and the brain, and quickening the reflexes. Chronic stress in response to a psychosocial stressor, such as a loved one's illness, is distinctly less adaptive; it can have deleterious effects on blood pressure, immune function, memory, and mood. Chronic stress in the form of post-traumatic stress disorder (PTSD) appears to shrink the part of the brain called the hippocampus, which is responsible for memory processing. Although the exact mechanism of hippocampal damage is not yet clear, one hypothesis is that stress hormones impair the ability of hippocampal neurons to regenerate.[23] Bottom line: acute stress is adaptive; chronic stress appears maladaptive.

What is a key ingredient of chronic stress? Feeling out of control. We humans love to feel like we're in control, even when we're not. This is why we have developed superstitions, beliefs that explain why something happened to us so that we don't feel like things happen for arbitrary and unpredictable reasons. When a loved one is sick, we are definitely not in complete control, and that can result in enormous stress. The key to relieving that stress is to regain a sense of control in some arenas and relinquish the need for control of other aspects of the experience.

Laura could not control whether she had a flood in her laundry room. She chose to control who cleaned up the mess. She also exerted control in some smaller but still significant ways; for example, she chose to vent to a supportive friend. When overwhelmed by a stressful day, consciously choose to take care of yourself with small gestures. Listen to a favorite CD while driving on that frustrating errand. Take a five-minute break to talk to a friend. Schedule a massage for next week. Just knowing that hour of nurturing is coming up may help you feel you are handling things better.

---

23   Robert M. Sapolsky, *Monkeyluv: And Other Essays on Our Lives as Animals* (New York: Scribner, 2005).

CHAPTER 5
Discovering Opportunities

How does stress promote growth? By moving us out of our comfort zone, adversity forces us to find new ways of being. A loved one's illness may confront us with the need to slow down, intentionally foster gratitude, and develop deeper reserves of patience. At the same time, we may learn to recognize our limitations and accept our fallible human nature.

Personal Growth

When you are inspired by some great purpose...
dormant forces, faculties, and talents become alive,
and you discover yourself to be a greater person
by far than you ever dreamed yourself to be.
—PATANJALI

I'm not absolutely sure that pain is a necessary condition for growth, but I believe there may be some truth to that notion. Years ago I had a conversation with a friend that has stayed with me to this day. He argued that until you experience a life trauma or tragedy, you live on a simple plane and are unable to have a true understanding of gratitude or an opportunity to grow in a meaningful way. I remember thinking at the time that this friend was condescending and judgmental. Even though I hadn't suffered a particularly monumental loss or hardship at that point in my life, I felt that I knew how to appreciate my blessings and experience regular growth.

But now sometimes I wonder. Are there certain epiphanies that emerge only through struggle? Is there a state of illumination that we reach only by trudging through the darkness? Are there valuable lessons we can never access any other way?

Dealing with my husband's cancer turned me unequivocally into a grown-up. I was compelled to confront a life-or-death situation, provide leadership for my family, and rely on my capabilities at a level I had never before been forced to perform. Was I mature enough for my new life?

> *G showed me an essay she wrote. I was touched by her words that she admired her mom for "being so brave." I want to be brave for the kids and for Bill—and for myself. And positive and strong and normal. I want them to feel like, no matter what happens, we are still a family. We won't fall apart.*

It is true that we are shaped by adversity. Starting in infancy, we grow from opportunities to adapt to challenge and frustration. D. W. Winnicott, a psychoanalyst who developed object-relations theory, described the "good enough mother" as a parent who could meet the infant's needs so well most of the time that the infant could survive a certain amount of "optimal frustration" of those needs.[24] Through withstanding the frustration, the infant develops his or her autonomous sense of self. As the small child matures, greater opportunities for autonomy arise, and these help shape his or her self-esteem and competence.

---

24 D. W. Winnicott, "The Theory of the Parent-Infant Relationship," *The International Journal of Psychoanalysis*, 41, Nov-Dec (1960): 585-595.

Since human development continues throughout the life cycle, we continue to have opportunities to grow whenever we encounter difficulty. Every time we have a difficult interpersonal encounter, an experience of failure, or some other challenge, we get to choose how to respond. When we choose the same old way that didn't work so well the last time, we miss the opportunity to grow. When we try a new way, we increase our chance for success. Even if the new way doesn't work that well, examining its failure may help us figure out a better solution for the next time. The accrual of hundreds and thousands of these successes and failures leads to wisdom and maturity. If there were no challenges to face, we would experience no impetus for growth.

When it comes to facing new challenges, it may startle you to see the things you are capable of doing. I have always considered myself squeamish, and although I am a well-educated person, I stopped taking science after tenth grade. So my medical skills had been limited to taking my children's temperatures and administering Tylenol. However, like many people in a caregiving role, I surprised myself with how composed and competent I was when I assumed some duties way beyond my usual comfort level, such as draining the gravy-like fluid that repeatedly built up in Bill's chest wall. There was something gratifying about being able to help him in such a tangible and intimate way.

When you are dealing with illness, especially one that has thrown you into limbo, it can feel like an accomplishment just to survive, to get out of bed in the morning, and to get through the day. But at some point, it might occur to you that this chapter of your life may last for a while, even a long time, and you will be cheating yourself if your life becomes about only this particular set of circumstances.

Are there things you can learn? Ways you can grow? Can you build your own character strengths to become the finest self you can possibly be throughout this period and beyond?

Regardless of the ultimate outcome, most of us will be forever changed by this experience. We will have new insights into virtues such as courage, humility, compassion, strength, and selflessness. And this is a silver lining.

Writer Isabel Allende described how she took care of her twenty-eight-year-old daughter, who became ill and fell into a coma, for a year before she died. In recounting how that period of caretaking gave her a chance to reflect on her beliefs, she wrote, "Paralyzed and silent in her bed, my daughter taught me a lesson that is now my mantra: you only have what you give. It's by spending yourself that you become rich." [25]

I am not suggesting that we approach this time merely in a self-focused way, reframing the situation to make it about our own opportunities as caregivers. This period of limbo is about our loved one with the illness, but it is *also* about us. It is about how we can grow and rise to the occasion. And as Allende expresses, it is about truly experiencing how giving and giving again can create intensely deep connections with others and provide our lives with ultimate meaning.

There is nothing wrong with feeling good about yourself when you accomplish a task or handle a situation well. In some cases, such as caring for someone with dementia or another cognitive disorder, you may be the only one around who can appreciate what you are doing. I remember that when one of my children studied character development in elementary school, she was taught that character is who you are and what you do "even when no one is watching." Our own moral compass, our own sense of satisfaction, our own self-distributed reward, may be the only recognition we get for many of the things we do. As Allende articulates, not only can our own giving impact us positively, but it also may bring us to a place where we access our truest beliefs and values. When we view our challenging situation in only a negative light, we lose the inherent potential to take measure of our lives and transform ourselves.

---

25 Jay Allison and Dan Gediman, eds., *This I Believe: The Personal Philosophies of Remarkable Men and Women* (New York: H. Holt, 2006), 14.

Our difficult feelings and thoughts are part of who we are. When we dismiss distressing beliefs and feelings as irrational, we choose to elevate the tidy but perhaps constricting structure of rationality over the growth that may occur by engaging those thoughts and emotions that are uncomfortable. We reject the difficult in favor of the easy. Throughout history, great science and art have been produced by people who have dared to face and derive inspiration from the chaos. Living in limbo makes us acutely aware that our time on this earth is finite, and therefore, our opportunities must be discovered and executed.

Accepting Who You Are

If you aren't in over your head, how do you know how tall you are?
—T. S. ELIOT

Even with something this huge going on in my life, it doesn't protect me or stop all of the other problems from still presenting themselves, bothering and distracting me. Life keeps going on, and as the new problems pop up, all of the old ones continue. And though in many ways I've got beyond certain petty things, in some ways I haven't.

Although this section of the book focuses on finding those moments of inspiration in the caregiving process, I must certainly acknowledge that there are many, many times when we feel anything but transcendent and virtuous. We may even feel guilty when trivial annoyances still get under our skin, when we believe that, despite the incentive to grow, we feel like the same average people we were before.

While countless books tell us how to find the blessings in the crises we face, people with illnesses and their caregivers often bristle at what they perceive to be rose-colored platitudes. Not everyone feels positively transformed by the process of dealing with illness; we don't all learn profound life lessons. Moreover, most motivational books I have encountered about illness have been written for the benefit of the patient, not for the support person. The way you, as caregiver, experience the situation may differ dramatically from your loved one's experience.

One day when Bill was in treatment, I had a minor squabble with one of my children—the type that occurs routinely throughout American households on a daily basis. After it was resolved, however, I felt an overwhelming sense of regret about the interaction. In a disproportionately harsh self-recrimination, I reasoned that I was now a person who should be *above* petty arguments, given the perspective my situation should afford me. After several other instances of overly self-critical assessments of insignificant incidents, I came to realize that my new life circumstances did not impose a requirement that I must now feel and behave with some sort of enlightened transcendence at all times.

There are opportunities for us even when this period in our lives does not prove to be a source of aspiration or inspiration. It can be a time when we find and appreciate the qualities that make us who we are even if they aren't exemplary, because regardless of what happens to us and how we respond, we remain regular, imperfect people. We all have those moments we later lament when we react in frustration or anger, but even those times can be valuable, because they sharpen our ability to acknowledge that we are only human. By experiencing times where we respond "badly," we are forced to accept our shortcomings as part of our selves. Our humility can release us from the burden of being perfect, creating an opportunity for liberation and tranquility.

Over time we can learn to be gentle and accepting of ourselves. This period may give us a chance to develop qualities to which we have always aspired, but it will also be a time when we may feel we have fallen short of our own or others' expectations. It is best to stay away from value judgments and accept our foibles along with our achievements. Having a loved one with a serious illness does not compel us to become superhuman. This is a time to cultivate self-compassion.

The people I know who have handled a loved one's illness with genuine grace tend to have two things in common: a healthy sense of humor and a willingness to acknowledge their mistakes. When something does not go well, rather than getting bogged down in guilt or hopelessness, these people find a way to step back from their momentary "failure" and try again a different way.

For example, a mother caring for a child with cancer at home felt terribly guilty when she accidentally hit her son with her handbag as they were both getting into the car, bumping him right where his indwelling chemotherapy catheter was located. After a wave of guilt washed over her, she used her humor and wit to recover from the event and to prevent its recurrence. She invented a silly little "Handbag Song" that prompted her to be more mindful of her movements when getting into and out of cars and that the family cheerfully adopted as a mood changer any time someone did something careless.

We are each imperfect and make mistakes, even when everything is going smoothly. Only a Stepford Wife would keep her cool throughout something as stressful as a prolonged illness. I have found that the best way to handle my mistakes is to acknowledge them and then find a way to repair the problem. If you find yourself in the middle of an argument with someone you care about, you might try to interrupt it by saying, "This isn't going well. Let's start over from the beginning." Then start the conversation from the top, trying to do a better job of listening to the other person and communicating what you want.

Appreciating What Is Good

> *No one is as capable of gratitude as one who*
> *has emerged from the kingdom of night.*
> —Elie Wiesel

I regret that up until now, I have lived with a complacency that results from a lack of urgency, a sense that my life would be like it is forever or for a very long time. I became lazy about my gratitude, postponing it, neglecting it.

Bittersweet. The bitter of having so much at stake. The sweet of having so much at stake. The price of having so much is also the reward.

Illness is nothing to idealize, and you won't find me in the camp that promotes the perspective that illness is a gift. However, I truly believe there are gifts to be found and blessings to be realized even when life seems grim and bleak. One of the wisest pieces of advice from my therapist was this: "You don't get to choose everything about your life. There are things you wouldn't choose but many that you would. Love the things that are right."

What are the gifts and blessings?

- The gift of living in the present
- The gift of family, close friends, and community
- The gift of modern medical treatment or good palliative care
- The gift of discovering your inner strengths
- The gift of selflessness
- The gift of devotion
- The gift of living with a higher purpose
- The gift of living with an intensity you have never before experienced
- The gift of appreciating what you do have

Although it may be one of the hardest things you have ever done, try to find as many moments as possible when you can experience pure enjoyment without the feeling of foreboding. Figure out a way to integrate gratitude into your life. In addition to the rewards you gain from your awareness of the blessings, you may also recover your energy and optimism, most helpful companions in this journey.

If the negatives are obstructing your ability to recognize the positives, make a mental, or even a written, list of everything that is good in your life. Make another list of the names of people or resources you feel you can count on for support. You might even carry these lists around with you in your wallet to look at when you feel overwhelmed.

I am writing this section while on an airplane traveling home to Denver from San Diego. We just experienced a gorgeous, sunny week on beaches and boardwalks in shorts and sandals. We are flying into a blizzard. Everyone in my family has been bemoaning the change in conditions we are about to experience. Just now the flight attendant announced in a perky voice, "Welcome to winter!" Yes, there is much to appreciate: The skiers on our flight will have excellent conditions. The home-for-the-holiday types will have a white Christmas. Many of the children aboard will see their first snow. Love what is right.

When you are looking for the good things, it may be necessary to redefine for yourself what is meant by "good." For example, as much as we wanted CT scans to show improvement or less disease, our doctor considered no change to be good, even great. A stable (even if not better) X-ray may be reason to celebrate.

Feeling good is good. Having an appetite is good. Walking around the block twice is good. Recognizing the grandchildren is good. Just like hope, how you view good may change over time. Love what is good.

Sometimes Bill or I would find ourselves pointing out the ways we were lucky. It seemed like a funny word to use when overall we felt quite unlucky about the situation. But still, we would say the following:

- "We're lucky we have a good doctor" (or "good insurance" or "a good support system").
- "We're lucky there are new treatments in the pipeline."
- "We're lucky it hasn't spread to the other lung."
- "We're lucky there haven't been any bad side effects."
- "We're lucky we were able to take this trip."

Although real luck would have been not getting the illness in the first place, I did find myself reflecting on the good luck amid the bad. There is usually something you can find that is positive. It may sound odd, but I did find consolation in thinking about the ways it could have been worse. And if you have as active an imagination as I do, it will be easy to come up with them. Our neighbor's friend, younger than Bill, had a completely unexpected fatal heart attack. I felt lucky. At least we had a chance.

> The more you look for the good, the more you'll notice it. This is a powerful way to combat demoralization and despair. Our minds are wired to collect information that confirms our beliefs and expectations. For example, when a woman is trying to get pregnant, she may have the impression that pregnant women are everywhere. In reality, pregnant women are as prevalent as they were the year before, but since now the woman's mind registers them as important data, she notices them more.

> We can choose to notice information that confirms our positive expectations or our negative ones. Laura and Bill were intent on noticing the ways in which they were lucky. The more examples they could find of their luck, the more information they had to bolster their hope and belief that they were going to get lucky with a cure. Maintaining such positive hope and belief helps to reinforce a positive mood and health-promoting behaviors. Had Bill focused instead on pessimistic stories that confirmed his worst fears, his mood may have been depressed, and he might have felt hopeless or helpless. These feelings, in turn, may have interfered with his decision to exercise, eat a healthy diet, and search for new medical treatments.

Patience and Perspective

When your life is filled with the desire to see the
holiness in everyday life, something magical happens:
ordinary life becomes extraordinary, and the very
process of life begins to nourish your soul.
—RABBI HAROLD KUSHNER

In many ways, I feel more conscious of receiving benefit from how pro-
found my life is right now. As I improve my ability to manage my fears,
I am able to experience my life in a deeper, more productive way and to
become a person who can do that more often in order to preserve our happy
memories and continue to make more.

When Bill became sick, I realized it was more important than ever to be aware of and grateful for the everyday moments of contentment. Times I might previously have categorized as uneventful or even dull I now elevated to precious in their ordinariness. So often we are on the lookout for whatever is bigger, better, faster, or finer as our reliable possessions get quickly outmoded for something substantially more exciting. Too often we are apt to view our lives in the same way. Until crisis occurs. Then we want to scurry back to the good, old days that we suddenly view with wistful appreciation. Bringing that grateful consciousness to our mundane moments helps us find the blessings and beauty in things we formerly might have taken for granted.

Years ago I was in a playgroup with several other mothers of preschoolers. As irony would have it, the youngest, most health conscious of us all was abruptly diagnosed with advanced cancer. Her illness progressed quickly, and before long, she was too sick to do much except rest in her apartment. Friends organized to help take care of her three young daughters while her husband finished his medical residency.

I will never forget when my friend told me that something she missed the most was shopping for and making lunches for her kids. Now, if there was one thing that every mother I knew complained about universally, it was packing lunches for their children. I was always quick to participate in conversations about the hassle of making lunch: thinking of things the kids would eat, keeping track of who likes and hates what, the craziness of the morning scramble, the terrible waste of uneaten food—it could go on and on.

However, after that chat with my friend, I'm pretty sure I never complained about making school lunches again. I became conscious of appreciating that I had the energy and health to go to the store and fill my basket with food my children would enjoy and pack three individualized lunches that they would open when we were all involved in our separate days. I thought about how my morning effort would touch my kids several hours later. It was a way I could stay connected to them. Finding the blessing in this mundane chore was a gift I received from my friend. If not for that conversation, I'm sure I would still view making lunch as a thankless burden.

Another place I felt I gained perspective was in facing the small aggravations in life that continued to occur. Rather than losing patience with them, I became much better at denying them access to my consciousness, where they previously had enjoyed free reign. I knew I needed to reserve my mental bandwidth for more important thoughts and concerns.

Experiences such as waiting an inexplicably long time in a line or having a restaurant order botched were revealed to me as small problems. I found that once I was dealing with a really big problem, my tolerance for the smaller ones increased exponentially. It surprised me that rather than adding to my stress, the everyday annoyances actually lowered it, because they gave me perspective. I looked for the humor in outrageous behaviors. I appreciated tiny crises that I could solve effortlessly. Of course I did not want to become one of those individuals who act superior or smug in their status as people with "real" problems, but dealing with a major challenge ironically made certain parts of my life easier.

Another place where I found an opportunity for self-improvement was in developing the art of patience. Being in limbo, I felt that I had to tolerate so much uncertainty, and somehow I had no choice other than to sit back and be patient. Is the treatment working? Is the disease progressing? I didn't know and realized I might not know for a while. Meanwhile, I had to figure out a way to live my life while anticipating the one piece of information that mattered the most to me. I postponed getting lunch or finding a receptive spot for a cell-phone call for hours, because I didn't know if the doctor might come by the hospital room. I sat in waiting rooms, so aptly named for the heroic periods people spend on pins and needles awaiting news that might provide renewed hope or utter devastation.

As caregivers, it can be incredibly frustrating that so much about our loved one's condition is outside the scope of our control. Patience is a proverbial virtue, and yet it may run counter to every instinct we have. Without it, however, we are in for severe aggravation. It will serve you well to cultivate this trait, an important tool for your continuing voyage.

How does one cultivate patience? The frenetic pace of modern life encourages us to use every minute for some kind of productive activity. Relaxation is almost sinful, considered to be a waste of time. If you have to wait, you have the choice between doing it in an impatient, stressed-out manner or doing it with an intentionally relaxed attitude. The more a person learns to slow down and relax, the easier it becomes.

An attitude of patience may be easier to adopt in short-term situations, like waiting longer than expected in the doctor's office, which is possible to do when you and your loved one each have brought along something good to read or some knitting or an iPod with favorite music and a recently downloaded podcast. Now the unexpectedly long wait is an opportunity to linger over a pleasant activity.

Patience with waiting for longer periods, especially when the time frame for the wait is uncertain, is more challenging and is at the root of the limbo experience. For example, if your loved one has hepatitis B and is undergoing treatment with interferon, an immune modulator that causes a chronic flu-like state, you will have to be patient with months of uncertainty. Even the duration of the treatment is uncertain, contingent on the response after four to six months, depending on the treatment protocol.

Maintaining patience over long and undefined periods of time is a practice that draws on the skills discussed elsewhere in this book: mindfulness, trust, flexibility, and courage. If you set your mind to cultivating and responding with patience, then you will have repeated opportunities to mindfully notice where and when impatience appears and then to adjust your response.

If at month four of interferon, the doctor determines that another four-month course is required, after which, "We'll see," your initial response might be, "I can't do this for another four months!" Remind yourself that you are not the person receiving the interferon injections and experiencing the relentless flu-like symptoms. Intentionally re-frame your response so that you can recapture patience. Can you be patient for another week? Another day? Break it down to something you can handle, and just practice patience for that interval. Like any other skill, patience improves with intentional repetition.

An exercise for building patience begins with noticing the rising tension of impatience as early in its development as possible. Our reactivity in impatience comes from seeing *ourselves* in the center of the situation and focusing on the impact it has on *us*. Try to widen the space between rising impatience and losing your cool by ex-panding your perspective of the situation. If you feel you're waiting too long for an appointment and notice yourself growing testy with the clinic staff, it may help to imagine that the doctor is dealing with an emergency even greater than your own. If you feel your ire rising as you wait on hold for too long with an insurance company and feel tempted to explode on the customer-service agent, imagine that person's job, caught between frustrated customers and a demand-ing corporate environment. The agent probably is doing the best he or she can and may feel as frustrated as you.

Restructuring Your Priorities

Live as if you were to die tomorrow.
Learn as if you were to live forever.
—MAHATMA GANDHI

As much as I feel that I have lost control of my life, I also feel that I have gained control in small ways. If I could step back and observe myself, one of the things that would be most fascinating to me is how much and how quickly I have adjusted my priorities. It is so liberating to decline activities that are merely obligations. I can't do obligations right now.

A positive by-product of caring for a loved one with a serious illness is the opportunity (and necessity) to prioritize what is truly important. It is a chance to say no to all the things that aren't meaningful. Once I had given myself the permission to choose how I spent my time and with whom, I realized how many hours and how much energy I normally devoted to activities that I felt compelled to do but that could really fall into the category of unnecessary busywork.

At a time when I felt I had no control over so many circumstances in my life, I looked for and found the places where I could assert some control. If I had to skip some activities or cut back on my compulsion to volunteer when no one else was stepping forward, I was confident that people would understand when I had to pull back from certain commitments that were more in the optional category. Making deliberate choices about how I would spend my time was a new and empowering concept for me.

In our youth, we often measure our social success by the quantity of our friends. We feel secure if we have a lot of people in our community repertoire. But many of them are very casual acquaintances, and as we age, we realize that true significance lies in the depth of our relationships, in their quality. Especially when we are going through a period in which we have a limited amount of personal resources, we need to allow ourselves to choose consciously where we put our energy. Being in crisis affords us the motive and opportunity to consider our connections and focus on the ones that are most nurturing and fulfilling.

Developing awareness and prioritizing our activities can open us to an enhanced quality of life. We have the opportunity for growth and self-actualization that we never may have previously emphasized. In the past, we may have found it easy to tend indiscriminately to everything on the to-do list, like getting the car washed or having a jacket altered. Of course, many of our day-to-day chores still need to get done, but maybe there are some that don't. This is where we can begin to restructure. (How important is a clean car or one more jacket in the closet? Maybe not very.)

The game of Jenga is a tangible example of how we can thoughtfully remove the pieces that don't matter so much. A tower of blocks is built, and the players take turns removing pieces that won't topple the structure. We look for those blocks on which the stability of the whole structure is not dependent. These are the low-hanging fruit. This game can be a metaphor for our lives: can we discover how to pull out those the nonessential pieces and set them aside?

> In our fast-paced society, almost all of us are doing too much. We think we are masters of multitasking, but that is not necessarily an achievement. Imaging studies of the brains of people engaged in multitasking show that rather than attending to several tasks at a time, the brain is shifting rapidly back and forth from one task to another, which actually decreases efficiency and increases the chance for error. [26]

> The most important task right now is taking care of your loved one. While you are doing that, try not to distract yourself with other activities. Yes, the laundry needs to get done, but if your loved one needs you to sit with him or her for a bit, the laundry can wait.

---

26 Summer Allen, "The Multitasking Mind," BrainFacts.org, 9 October 2013, http://www.brainfacts.org/Sensing-Thinking-Behaving/Awareness-and-Attention/Articles/2013/The-Multitasking-Mind.

In medical school, we are taught that if you sit down with a patient, the patient perceives that you are spending more time and paying better attention than if you remain standing. Even in a busy clinic, where the temptation is to look at the computer and write the note at the same time the patient is talking, doctors who take the first few minutes to sit facing the patient, listening and asking questions, have a superior bedside manner and are really no less efficient than their less attentive colleagues. By listening with full attention, the physician actually helps patients express their concerns more effectively, and the problem can be addressed more efficiently.

Why wouldn't a similar principle apply in all of our lives? It makes sense that if you give any task your full, undivided attention, you'll accomplish it faster and with fewer errors.

Treasuring Time with Your Loved One

There is no remedy for love but to love more.
—HENRY DAVID THOREAU

Bill will be walking in the door tonight, and I have that. I know that I have him today. That's all I know. And though it hurts to think that's all I can know, in reality, it's all I ever could know.

As mentioned previously, when you are living your life with an urgency you haven't before experienced, it can be quite striking how your priorities may change. Before he was sick, my time alone with Bill and our time alone as a family had been relegated to secondary status. Other engagements and opportunities usually came first, because we could always be together another time. But when you are in a position where time feels of the essence, you worship and covet your times with your loved one. They no longer play second fiddle.

One of the challenges you may face is when to splurge and when to be conservative. Although you can't live your life constantly planning "the last trip," your loved one may have a condition that makes it more likely that future vacations are questionable. This is the dilemma: If it is the last trip, you may want to indulge more than usual to make it special. But if it isn't, can you afford to spend your money on something more extravagant than you would under any other circumstances? Living in limbo forces you to analyze such situations carefully.

We took a family cruise to the Baltic that in the past we wouldn't have considered economically practical for us. But we wanted something especially memorable "just in case." As soon as we departed, we knew it was positively the right decision for us: ten glorious days of being together as a family. Cancer was not on board with us. With Bill between treatments, we didn't even have to think about his illness for one minute. Four thousand people on the ship, and not one of them knew our secret. We just looked like any other happy family enjoying a special vacation. We visited seven countries and had dessert at every meal. There was no question that, for us, the big dip into our savings was worth every penny and then some.

Of course, financial realities may work in the other direction. If you or your loved one are unable to work, you may find yourself buckling down more than ever. Splurging on a new car or a fancy vacation may be counter to your well-being. Look to find enjoyable things to do that are economical. Have game night at home with a big pot of spaghetti. Go to a discount movie. Take a walk through a nearby park or around the neighborhood. What is important is spending time together. If it turns out that your loved one ends up living another thirty years, you may find that you have created a more engaged connection than you would have had otherwise.

Over the course of the first few months following Bill's diagnosis, several family members and friends came from out of town to visit, including a college buddy of Bill's whom I had never met, even though we both had heard so much about each other over the years. A gift of living in limbo is the way that long-delayed intentions tend to come to the top of the list.

Another opportunity lies in having conversations that might not have been initiated but for the illness. Two friends of mine have recently lost their mothers, and both specifically mentioned how much they learned in the hours of bedside sitting. Tidbits about their mothers' or their own child-hoods, family secrets and scandals, hopes, dreams, and life philosophies were remembered or revealed. Both friends described these end-of-life in-teractions as among the most precious in the entire lifetime of their moth-er-daughter relationships.

And then there is the privilege of caregiving. At the risk of sounding as though I'm attempting to romanticize what can be an extremely difficult—if not heartbreaking—situation, I would be remiss if I didn't explain the sense I often had that what I did for Bill was meaningful and important. The comfort I was able to provide gave me a purpose that felt extremely significant and impactful. It was a role I alone was able to fulfill.

I think about when my children were little and would suffer a minor injury. As is the custom in many families, our ritual was for me to deliver a kiss to the boo-boo, making it all better. And most of the time it worked! What was that about? My lips applied to a bump or scrape were of no therapeutic benefit other than psychological. But somehow my presence and my action had power that was actually effective. Moreover, it had to be me. If another adult had delivered the exact same service, the magic effect of the cure would not have occurred.

Similar minor miracles happened frequently with Bill, and I was grate-ful when I managed to give him exactly what he needed when he needed it—whether it was a massage, a hearty laugh, or a good meal. One summer evening postchemo, he was feeling dispirited. My suggestion of taking a spur-of-the-moment drive to the foothills turned out to hit the spot for him perfectly.

It is certainly the case that caregiving may involve tasks that are difficult or unpleasant. In such circumstances, the duties might not feel like such a privilege. Still, it helps to focus on the relief and comfort you are able to provide to your loved one, to consider the unique role that you alone may perform during his time of hardship.

Resolving Broken Relationships

Life appears to me too short to be spent in
nursing animosity or registering wrongs.
—CHARLOTTE BRONTË

When a person is reevaluating his or her priorities, previously forsaken or postponed tasks, such as healing a broken relationship or dealing with unfinished business with a family member or friend, may come to the top of the list. A person with a new diagnosis may feel the motivation or even urgency to attempt reconciliations. Outreaching in this situation has the potential to have an extremely gratifying and meaningful outcome. It also has the risk of resulting in disappointment and renewed sorrow.

Sometimes connections that have soured or drifted are amenable to healing; illness can provide the perfect motive and opportunity to renew old bonds. We all know stories of estranged parents and children who have reconciled, distant siblings who have rekindled their bond, old friends who have rediscovered one another. The specter of illness can provide the incentive or even the excuse to reach out and let bygones be bygones. The prospect of losing a family member or formerly valued friend can lead people to realize that if they don't make an effort now, they may not have another opportunity to do so.

As caregiver or support person to someone with an illness, you may find yourself in a position to initiate or facilitate such an encounter. The success or failure of your effort may be unpredictable, so calibrate your and your loved one's expectations for the possibility of disappointment as well as for a satisfying outcome.

While some rifts may be candidates for mending, a bad relationship or situation in your life may be intransigent. Some estrangements are not amenable to healing, so you and your loved one may have to find a way to resolve that internally. Some people find peace through their own spirituality or merely by an acknowledgment that you have done what you can and are unable to devote any more energy to the problem. Maybe there is an alternative resolution that you can find through writing a letter (which you may or may not send), journaling, or visualization.

Sometimes the person with whom you or your loved one has unresolved issues isn't even available. He may be ill or deceased. He may be someone you lost track of many years ago. Even so, your loved one may feel the need to find some closure in the difficult or lost relationship. Maybe there is an indirect way to achieve this resolution. A technique from Gestalt therapy is using an empty chair to represent the other person. You can imagine that person sitting in the chair and then express yourself as though he is there. You can even then sit in the chair and imagine what he might say back to you.

This is a good time to let go of emotions that do nothing but weigh you down, such as guilt, resentment, regret, or jealousy. Find the healing power in intense, positive relationships; in expressions of love and gratitude; and in discovering your own assets. As you let go of petty problems, work on developing your own inner peace and equanimity. Dig deeper, if necessary.

CHAPTER 6

Interacting with Others

Responding to a loved one's illness is challenging enough without adding the stress of interacting with well-meaning but occasionally insensitive others. This is a time when you need support, and you may have to be quite explicit about what that entails. When people around you fall short of your expectations, it may help to discern what aspect of that interaction you are able to modify and what you must let go of and forgive.

Making Connections

> *Not knowing when the dawn will come, I open every door.*
> —EMILY DICKINSON

Facing a challenging new chapter in life can lead you to create bonds with others who have handled similar situations or other significant adversities. During some of the most testing times in my life, I have sensed a special connection with certain people with whom I hadn't previously felt close. Sometimes it has been expressed; other times, it has been tacit. But in either case, we mutually find a way to acknowledge being or having been there. The connection may be as simple as a feeling or an intuition. It can be with a close friend or a virtual stranger.

It is important to remember that while someone may have been through a similar situation, she may not have reacted the way you will react. It also does not necessarily mean that she will be helpful to you. On some occasions, I found myself with an acquaintance who made me feel worse rather than better, forcing me to figure out how to extricate myself from an upsetting situation.

We have all had our own traumas, or we will. You can't get out of this life unscathed. After Bill's diagnosis, when I made those first few shell-shocked trips to the grocery store, I had the typical thoughts so many people describe: Why does everyone seem so nonchalant when the world is obviously falling apart? It seemed like I was this ill-fated person alone in a sea of people who didn't have troubles. But the closer I looked, I could see pain and grief in others' faces. Most people have their own hardships. Some are silent or unacknowledged, like the inability to get pregnant, a troubled child, a family member with a mental illness, or a miserable marriage. It became clear to me that I wasn't the only one walking around the store in a daze.

In talking to other people during times of life crisis, many mention the ubiquitous grocery-store experience. It is the universal venue in which we tend to encounter that strange out-of-body sensation of being a changed person in the land of regular people. Maybe it is because nothing is more routine and necessary than trips to the store. Even though others may offer to run these errands for you, you can't escape the need to stop there for a prescription, a household item, or the one item your loved one thinks he can actually eat. The grocery store is static, unflappable. It offers reassurance in its familiarity and dependability. You can get what you need, and you know just where to find it.

The late-night straggling shoppers were the ones with whom I had a wordless connection. The women at the store at 9:30 or 10:30 buying diapers,

Depends, Ensure, soup, Jell-O, medicines—I knew they all had stories. I found myself making eye contact with them, all weary travelers on our own individual roads. It actually gave me comfort to imagine I had company in the hardships of life with these total strangers.

The Buddhist greeting "Namaste" means "The spark of the divine in me recognizes the spark of the divine in you." We usually think of the spark of the divine as love or holiness or goodness. It is equally possible for the spark of the divine to be compassion or even suffering. The Tibetan Buddhist deity Avalokiteshvara is depicted with eleven heads and a thousand arms; each of his thousand hands has an eye in the center of its palm. The Avalokiteshvara Buddha, the deity of compassion, uses his thousand eyes to see all the suffering in the world.[27]

When we connect to others through recognition of one another's suffering, we are embracing them and ourselves with compassion. There is no need to solve other people's problems, no need to give advice. Sometimes the healing we offer is merely in our listening to and acknowledging another person's pain. The words "I'm so sorry. What you're going through sounds really hard" are soothing, because they are validating. Witnessing another person's hardship or having our struggle witnessed is often enough.

Things People Say

Sweet mercy is nobility's true badge.
—SHAKESPEARE

I know people only mean well and are concerned. And I have been conscious of not passing judgment about what they say or don't say.

---

27   Min Bahadur Shakya, "Legends of 1000 Armed Avalokiteshvara," *Buddhist Himalaya: A Journal of Nagarjuna Institute of Exact Methods* 2, no. 1/2 (1989), http://buddhism.lib.ntu.edu.tw/FULLTEXT/JR-BH/bh117498.htm.

But I also know that they hear "advanced lung cancer," and it has death sentence written all over it. People can't help but react to that. Yet there are those who truly give messages of hope, who focus on all of the advances being made in treatment. I find myself lapping up those words like a thirsty puppy and replaying them over and over in my mind.

At first I was astounded by some of the things people said to me, which left me speechless. I found it disheartening when a few folks were quick to write Bill off completely as a hopeless case. A curiously large number of people told me about others they had known who had died of the same cancer. Many prematurely jumped to the worst-case scenario: "At least you'll have time to prepare, unlike my friend whose husband was killed in a car accident." "My college roommate was also widowed in her forties, when her husband was killed in the World Trade Center." "I can give you the name of an excellent grief group for children who have lost a parent."

I wanted to put my hands on these people's shoulders, shake them, and call out, "Bill is still alive!"

How could I integrate all this? Bill wasn't killed in an accident or during the September 11 attacks; our children still had both parents. My husband was doing well and feeling fine, but some people were already giving me condolences on what they saw as his inevitable fate. I found myself on the defensive, not wanting to buy into others' assertions that we were doomed.

Other uncomfortable conversations were the ones that started with something like "I don't know how you do it. I could never handle something like this" or "You're so amazing. I would be such a mess."

I know I was particularly vulnerable and possibly irrational, but even though these comments were clearly meant to be compliments, I often heard them as accusations (as in, "How can you be so calm and collected when your husband is so sick?"). In my fragile state of mind, I would interpret this praise as an allegation that something was wrong with me. If other people assumed they wouldn't react the way I did, then was I abnormal?

When people insisted they "could never handle it," I would feel (again, probably illogically) that the comment was given as an explanation of why this type of thing had happened to me, not them—because I could handle it, and they couldn't. But the fact was that I felt I didn't have a choice.

When people said, "I don't know how you can deal with this," I would want to cry out, "What is the alternative?" I suppose I could have stayed in bed with the covers over my head, but with three kids, a job, and a husband with a serious illness, this didn't seem to be a viable option. I believe the vast majority of people can deal with adversity, even if they assume they can't.

The old adage "God doesn't give you more than you can handle" felt like another backhanded compliment. This comment and variations on it made me feel that I had somehow brought the situation on myself by being so strong that God was compelled to think up something that would be challenging enough for me.

Not everyone handles adversity the same way. Not everyone is able to handle it in a functional way. It is common and normal to be listless, to feel paralyzed, and to lack optimism and motivation. I experienced mornings when I stayed in my bed for a long time after I was awake, unable to face my world. I spent some afternoons with my face buried in my pillow, drenched in weepy disbelief and heartache. There were hours at my desk at work where I accomplished nothing but obsessive worrying. Those were the times people rarely saw. They saw me as doing well, and my tendency to sometimes hear their kind words as insults most likely reflected my own insecurity about how I should feel and act in the alien territory that was now my life.

Ultimately the best way for me to handle comments that made me feel hurt or uncomfortable was to realize the following: 1) many people felt awkward and didn't know what to say; 2) no one was mean or malicious; and 3) different things are helpful to different people. These may seem like obvious observations, but when you are on the receiving end of what feels like a thoughtless comment, it helps to keep this perspective: people don't want to hurt you, but they also may be ill at ease.

In the same way I needed to learn to be generous with myself and my own capabilities, I needed likewise to be generous with others. The concern shown to us by our friends and family was always genuine and so often above and beyond our wildest expectations. I had to remind myself of the many times in my life when I fretted that I had said the wrong thing, when I may have added salt to a wound rather than relieved it. It would be hypocritical for me to judge people more harshly than I would have hoped to be judged in similar situations.

> In their eagerness to be helpful, family members, friends, and co-workers sometimes offer unwelcome advice or outright criticism. Even people with great self-confidence are not always secure enough in their decisions about how they are handling things to be able to politely shrug off unharmonious comments. Well-intentioned advice that does not support your path in dealing with an illness can be very unsettling and can raise fear, doubt, guilt, and confusion. It may also elicit anger at the person who offered the advice. None of this is useful to you, and it may divert your attention and energy while you try to sort through your reactions.
>
> One helpful strategy for managing inadvertently unsupportive comments is to consider the source. In its common use, this phrase has a pejorative connotation, as in, "Well, of course the comment was abrasive; the person who made it is a jerk." While this may make you feel a little better, it leaves you with negative

feelings toward the person, which may damage a relationship you want to keep. By "consider the source," I mean to spend a little time thinking about the person who made the comment. Who is he? What are his values? What do you know about his background and current life? In the context of that person's life and values, does the comment make more sense?

The father of one of my patients told her she was "coddling" her son, who had repeatedly injured his knees in sports. The father offered the comment when he learned that the teenage boy was not required to do chores. Initially, my patient felt criticized and insecure. Was she a bad mother? Was she encouraging excessive dependency in her son? Next came anger: "How dare he criticize me? He has no idea what it's like to watch your son endure multiple orthopedic surgeries!"

With further reflection, she realized that her father, raised on a ranch during the Depression, had had a very different childhood. He had performed chores as far back as he could remember and was proud of it. Independence, physical strength, and stoicism were his highest values. With this in mind, my patient was able to have more compassion for her father, realizing he was afraid for his grandson because of his injured legs and perhaps was also envious of his grandson's more comfortable, urban, middle-class existence.

My patient was able to see that her father's values were not the same as hers; she prized connectedness, emotional warmth, and a nurturing style of parenting. By taking the time to deeply consider the source of her father's unsupportive comment, she was able to feel closer to her father, who was clearly trying to impart helpful advice. Simultaneously she could comfortably reject his advice, because it was not congruent with her values about how to raise her child.

Accepting Others' Reactions

*Accept what people offer. Drink their
milkshakes. Take their love.*
—WALLY LAMB

It is not realistic or fair to expect everyone to match where you are, especially when your needs or expectations can be a moving target. My reactions to what people did or didn't do were more about me than about them. Giving people the benefit of the doubt is a virtue that was helpful for me to try to cultivate. Once I recognized that making assumptions about people and rushing to judgment only made me upset and distracted, I could see that by becoming more accepting in my thinking, I could keep my mind clear for the more important matters at hand.

Recognize that friends, family, coworkers, and neighbors have their own preconceptions about illness in general or about the specific diagnosis you and your loved one are confronting. They have their own life experiences, which may or may not be relevant to yours. People want to be empathic, but their idea about what is helpful might differ from yours. There were times when someone would act in a way that felt unkind or unthinking, but in almost every case, I knew that the best thing to do was to let it go and assume that person's heart was in the right place. It doesn't serve any purpose to dwell negatively on interactions you find disappointing. And it is always important to leave room for the possibility that your expectations were unreasonable or not clearly expressed. Our friends and family members do not convert into mind readers when we are feeling stressed and overwhelmed.

Letting go of negative emotions is easier to do when the problem is small, like when someone cut you off in traffic or failed to send a thank-you card for a gift, or similar minor infractions of social etiquette. We can all agree that there are better ways to use our energy than stewing about these kinds of mistakes. Often, just stating the problem to yourself or a close friend, acknowledging the negative feelings that resulted from the insult, and resolving to let it go is enough to do the trick.

It might sound like, "When Mary spent the night last weekend, I went out of my way to make her stay pleasant. It irks me that she didn't help out with any of the meals and didn't send a thank-you note. I really don't need to be taking care of other people right now, and I also don't want to expend the energy to deal with the conflict it would create if I confronted her about this. Next time she announces a visit, I'll tell her it's not a good time."

Often the resolution to do things differently next time brings a sense of relief; knowing you will protect yourself from a repetition helps dissolve the present feelings of resentment. There are some things one can't control, like whether a person cuts in front of you in line, but you can decide how to respond the next time it happens (will you say something or not?), thus gaining a small measure of control.

It's much more challenging to release resentment when it is a deep-seated feeling developed over years in your family of origin. Sometimes it is possible to have a heart-to-heart with the family member that permits healing. More often these conversations fall short of our expectations and become merely a rehashing of the same old grievances, leaving both people freshly hurt and resentful.

It may be more adaptive to acknowledge to yourself that the other person has certain behaviors or attitudes that have disappointed or hurt you, that you are powerless to change the other person, and that persisting in wanting the person to be different further dashes your hopes and wishes. In this case, it is not the other person who will change; it is your hopes and wishes that may need reevaluation. Admitting to yourself that the other person has limitations and forming more realistic expectations of your relationship is the path to leaving old resentments behind and freeing yourself from further injury.

Some people use the following exercise to facilitate releasing resentment.[28] Bring to mind a situation with another person that built resentment. Remember what happened and how it made you feel. Acknowledge and accept your feelings. Now try to imagine how the other person experienced the situation, replaying it from that person's point of view. What do you imagine the other person was feeling? Finally, imagine how the scenario might have gone differently if you had each understood what was driving the other person's behavior as it was happening.

This exercise allows you to rewrite the story as an omniscient narrator, a process that lifts you out of your personal, wounded feelings into a position of wisdom and understanding. By the end of the exercise, you may notice that you have more compassion for yourself and for the other person and that your resentment has diminished.

Diagram of Change in a Resentment Pathway

Situation: Your mother/sister/best friend did not call to ask how the much-anticipated visit with the new medical specialist went.
Your initial response: "She doesn't care. She has forgotten about me and my problems. She's only focused on herself."
Your feelings: Hurt, perhaps angry or alienated.
The other person's perspective as you imagine it: "I really want to know how the meeting with the specialist went today, but I'm reluctant to call. I don't want to add any extra responsibilities for my child/sister/friend. I'll wait for her to call me."

---

28 Adapted from Barbara Zilber, LCSW, cofounder of Elderfire, personal communication, 2012.

Your response after this exercise: "She is being consider-ate. She understands that I am overloaded, and she wants to be helpful."

Your feelings after this exercise: Relieved, perhaps closer or less alienated.

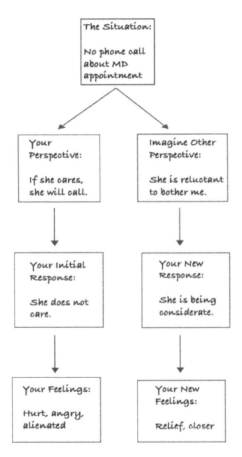

Handling Difficult Situations

There is a time for departure even
when there is no place to go.
—TENNESSEE WILLIAMS

There may be people in your life who, even when you are down, make you feel worse, those folks from whom you need distance or protection. In some cases, you may need to find a way to empower yourself (or a designated surrogate) to structure your interactions with the difficult person. If you feel incapable of discarding feelings of anger at or frustration with such a person, you may imagine yourself bracketing those emotions to deal with at a later time so that you aren't distracted from being present and available to your loved one and to yourself.

You may also encounter strangers who are rude and selfish. In these cases, try not to let their thoughtless comments ruin your day. For example, a woman who worked out at the same gym as Bill complained repeatedly about his heavy breathing while working out. Even after he explained to her that he had lung cancer, she maintained that she found it "gross" to have him working out near her. Although I was ready to follow him to the club and punch her out, he just ignored her and didn't let her spoil his morning routine.

Think about ways you might mitigate an awkward situation before it occurs. Anticipating things that might be uncomfortable can make your life a lot smoother. One time, when Bill's cough was particularly bad, we took a plane trip. This was shortly after it was discovered that a man with active tuberculosis had taken a commercial flight, potentially endangering everyone in his midst. I decided it would be best to try to preempt the alarm that Bill's cough might cause. I quietly notified the flight attendants and the people in the row in front of us that although Bill sounded terrible, he had lung cancer and was not contagious. People were sympathetic, and I could relax, knowing that my alerting people to Bill's condition had freed us as much as possible from being subject to anyone's fear, anger, or curiosity.

Keeping Family and Friends Informed

Be who you are and say what you feel, because those who
mind don't matter, and those who matter don't mind.
—Dr. Seuss

In this time of crisis, people will want to check in with you, and sometimes it adds to your stress when you feel that you need to answer every call, e-mail, or text. The fact is you may not have the time, energy, or desire to do so. It's OK. People will understand, and if they don't, you have to let go of the need to please everyone. Right from the start, I couldn't keep up with the phone calls, and I just had to assume people would cut us some slack. I was especially conscious of limiting my time on the phone in the evenings, because I felt that our kids were experiencing more trauma by hearing details of the latest appointment or disappointing news over and over again.

It is also completely acceptable and appropriate to leave a message that callers will hear explaining this directly, such as "We so appreciate your call and know that you will understand if we don't get back to you."

Keep in mind that people do care and are eager to find out what is happening. Bill chose to send blast e-mail updates when anything major occurred (positive or negative), and friends told us they appreciated receiving these. I know others who have used online care pages or personalized websites for this purpose. Our nephew-in-law wrote a wonderful blog to keep family and friends posted about our niece's cancer treatment. It provided the detail necessary to make all of us around the country feel up-to-date while greatly curtailing our instinct to pester them for every latest development.

You may be tempted, as I was, to pick and choose whom you want privy to certain information concerning your loved one's condition. Keep in mind that there is no way you can manage what people will say to one another. I found that I needed to feel comfortable enough with the information that I conveyed such that I wouldn't be distressed if it reached a wider audience than I had intended. We have all had the experience in which an e-mail we have written has been forwarded without our permission or knowledge to other recipients. We shudder in horror when we realize our words found their way to in-boxes we had never anticipated, and we learn the hard way that every e-mail should be written as though half the city might ultimately see it. The same is true of dispensing medical information.

Of course it can be very comforting to have one or more close confidants with whom you choose to freely share information. If you don't want your disclosures to be discussed with others, you may want to explicitly say so.

Some people ask a friend or family member to return calls or give updates on their behalf. It is important to give direction so that the intermediary is in sync with what you prefer. For example, a well-meaning relative may tell people not to visit when that is the exact opposite of your loved one's wishes. Or the point person might organize (or refuse) meals in contradiction to your desires. It is best to be clear about your needs and wishes in order to avoid misunderstandings and hurt feelings.

Be sensitive to the fact that the impact of a person's illness can be far-reaching. As much as I tended to focus on the effect of our experience on my family, I was certainly aware that Bill's diagnosis was taking a huge toll on others, personally and professionally. Recognizing this can make you more open to others' inquiries and genuine interest. In the workplace, your loved one's absence or diminished capacity may require that coworkers put in extra hours and effort to get the job done. Friends may struggle with their own vulnerability, mortality, and fear of losing an important relationship. The more informed they feel, the fewer assumptions they will make about your loved one's condition and how you are doing.

As I contemplated the fact that our immediate family's lives had been struck by a tornado, I had to keep in mind that those of our extended family and close friends had been hit, too. Even as they expressed their concern about us, they were also suffering deeply. Twisters often cut a wide swath, and the collateral damage can be greater than is readily apparent. Although I could not assume the responsibility of taking care of other people, an awareness of their pain gave me perspective and helped me move outside of myself.

I'm imagining now the dinner party we are having later this evening, a group we have hosted so many times that I can't even count them. How will it be different now? We are all different—every single one of our friends will sit at our table in a new way. I need to set the tone for our household—not of fear and despair but of hope and joy. Together we will begin to experience each other more consciously, maybe excruciatingly so.

CHAPTER 7
Taking Care of Yourself

The unremitting weight and responsibility of caring for someone with a serious medical condition take their toll. For example, studies have found that Alzheimer's caregivers have a rate of depression and demoralization three times higher than similar people not in this position. Physical health also tends to decline faster in caregivers. In addition to the exhausting tasks of supervising and performing daily activities for their loved one, caregivers often become socially isolated, unable to go out with friends and participate in their former pursuits. Clearly those of us taking care of people with illnesses or disabilities can be overcome with physical and mental exhaustion. Only by taking care of ourselves can we sustain the energy and strength to stay on duty.

Your Physical Care

> *To keep the body in good health is a duty...otherwise we*
> *shall not be able to keep our mind strong and clear.*
> —BUDDHA

How well do you take care of yourself? For many of us, our own health feels secondary, even insignificant, in the face of our loved one's serious condition, but nothing could be further from the truth. Our mental and physical well-being directly affects our ability to cope with the situation and, consequently, care for the person who is ill or disabled.

We all know to eat well, exercise regularly, and get some sunshine and adequate sleep. These tenets of a healthy lifestyle are even more critical when your energy and stamina are being tested to their limits. You may have to make an extra effort to accomplish these fundamentals.

For some of us, sleep comes easily as a welcome respite from our physical and emotional labors. For others, it mercilessly evades us even as we are shrouded in a blanket of fatigue. Attending to this deficit is a top priority, whether through relaxation exercises; cognitive-behavioral therapy and self-soothing techniques; or prescription medications, if necessary.

Promptly attend to any concerns about your own health. You need to be in your best possible shape to cope effectively with the demands you are facing. Be mindful of the strains on your physical condition as well as your mental health, but also be watchful for hypervigilance that might result from being overly watchful and anxious. Knowing that your loved one and other family members are relying on you may cause you to worry about every ache and pain you experience. Two days after Bill's diagnosis, I discovered a few tiny black spots on my fingers. Almost in a panic that I had developed melanoma, I was able to get the dermatologist's office to bypass a six-week waiting list to see me immediately. It turned out that I had developed some minuscule blood blisters that the compassionate doctor calmly showed me through a magnifying glass.

This preoccupation with small physical signs and symptoms is also known as medical-student syndrome.[29] In the first two years of medical school, while studying the presenting symptoms of scores of dreaded diseases, it is common for students to become anxious about their own minor physical anomalies. If a disease can present

29 R. Collier, "Imagined Syndromes Can Cause Real Problems for Medical Students," *Canadian Medical Association Journal* 178, no. 7 (2008): 820.

with any of twenty symptoms, a person is certain to have one or two of them at some point, especially when those symptoms are common.

Fatigue, lack of energy, weight gain or loss, and trouble with sleep are almost universal accompaniments to illness, but they are also the natural state of medical students. Immersed in studying pathology, the student becomes convinced that a raised scar is actually a nonpigmented melanoma, a tension headache is a sign of a brain tumor, or a racing heart rate during a verbal presentation to an intimidating attending physician is actually an indicator of underlying cardiac arrhythmia and impending death.

Over time medical students learn to relax their vigilance about their own bodies, and so can you. Remember to take good care of yourself and see a doctor if something feels wrong, but try to let go of anxiety about your health that may drive you to overfocus on minor and insignificant concerns about your body.

Nurturing Relationships

The friend who can be silent with us in a moment of despair or confusion, who can stay with us in an hour of grief and bereavement, who can tolerate not knowing... not healing, not curing...that is a friend who cares.
—HENRI NOUWEN

Research supports the generally accepted notion that social connectedness is extremely beneficial to a person's health and may be a predictor of how well a person with an illness fares. In *Open Heart: A Patient's Story of Life-Saving Medicine and Life-Giving Friendship*,[30] Jay Neugeboren describes how his deep friendships were key to his survival and recovery from

---

30 Jay Neugeboren, *Open Heart: A Patient's Story of Life-Saving Medicine and Life-Giving Friendship* (Boston: Houghton Mifflin, 2003).

emergency quintuple-bypass surgery. He cites many studies that show the importance of the emotional component of healing and its role in survival following serious illness. The impact of psychological healing is so strong that medical journals have published studies on the efficacy of placebos. Growing evidence indicates that placebos have significant benefit, ranging from 30 percent to 75 percent. No one can doubt the connection between a person's emotional well-being and his or her physical health.

I cannot overemphasize how important it is to have somebody or some buddies to talk to. Whether it's a good friend, a relative, a support group, or a therapist, try to find at least one person with whom you can share your feelings about this process.

Even though I tried to approach Bill's illness with optimism, I also had occasions when I wanted to have my misfortune validated. There were times when I needed my family and friends to acknowledge that Bill's diagnosis was terrible and unfair. It can be very isolating and lonely to go through this new and unfamiliar experience. I often felt disoriented and unanchored when I didn't have the touchstones I normally relied on to center me. In dealing with this foreign situation, it compounded the pain when I also felt insecure about my distressing emotions. This is when the special people in my life supported me through the discomfort and fear.

In a seemingly contradictory way, while I felt the desire for friends and family to recognize the struggle I was facing, I also found that I needed people to endorse and reinforce the hope I was trying to maintain. I imagine that my support people must have found this to be a demanding role: agree with me that this is horrible and senseless, but also build me up to believe things will be OK. If you find yourself in a similar situation, consider whether you are imposing overly burdensome expectations on your friends. It doesn't help you or them if you burn them out. Sometimes all you need is someone to witness all that you are doing and attest that it is important. But friends can't read your mind. If you are looking for a particular type of emotional support, figure out a gentle way to ask for it.

Pets can be another source of support and companionship. Many people find the devotion of their animals to be comforting and uplifting. The routines associated with caring for a pet help to keep life normal. About a year into Bill's illness, we adopted a new kitten, primarily for our young son. Miraculously, the cat seemed to know that his role was to attach to this particular child, giving him a sense of security and a nighttime bedmate.

Early in the AIDS epidemic, when there were few medications to combat the virus and most patients died from opportunistic infections or unusual malignancies, an important role for mental-health providers was bearing witness to the struggle people with AIDS were going through. Since then I've come to believe that most people yearn for a witness, someone to notice all they do. It feels wonderful to have one's efforts acknowledged, to be recognized for juggling multiple roles, for enduring hardship without much complaint, or for assuming extraordinary responsibility.

The Role of Community

Interdependence is and ought to be as much the ideal of man as self-sufficiency. Man is a social being.
—MOHANDAS GANDHI

When we feel part of a community or communities, that sense of belonging can be the most stabilizing and constant force in our lives. We can develop the identity of being a member of a particular fellowship of people in many different forums. Work; sports; school; religious congregations; athletic clubs; neighborhoods; professional associations; political committees; volunteer activities; or book, poker, card, or cooking groups—the list goes on and on. Community may be formal, such as a nonprofit board of directors, or it might be a casual girls-night-out group. Look to existing sources of community in which you might find outlets to distract you from your problems and people who can provide comfort and support to you.

If you are looking for a community of people who are likewise providing care to a loved one, for many diagnoses, there are organized support groups geared toward family members. Often the hospital or clinic can point you to such resources. Some people find these tremendously helpful; others can find them to be trauma inducing. Recognize that talking to friends and relatives of people who have a similar diagnosis as your loved one but who aren't doing well can be very upsetting.

A week or so after Bill's diagnosis, I went to a lung-cancer support group, and someone asked me if my husband was on oxygen "yet." At that point, the idea of oxygen hadn't even crossed my mind. I felt sick to my stomach the rest of the evening, as listening to other people's heartbreaking stories just made me more anxious, fearful, and sad. On the other hand, I have an acquaintance who found a great deal of comfort in a support group for parents of ill, premature newborns. This group and the cause provided so much meaning in her life that she ultimately made a career out of counseling parents with critically ill children. You are the only one who can determine whether attending a support group is right for you, and it is a decision that may change over time.

In today's world of social networking, many people turn to online chat rooms, Facebook, or other communities to find support, to meet others who are in similar situations, and to pursue connections that provide anonymity. While some people relish these avenues for communicating, we discuss in chapter 8 some of the pitfalls of using the Internet as an informational resource.

Illness is such a fundamental part of life, yet it is often ignored or shunted to the sidelines. In the past, most cultures included rituals that invited the community to participate in supporting the person who was ill, such as traditional Native American healing ceremonies and Hmong spirit-calling ceremonies. These rituals helped to place illness in the context of a person's social and spiritual life.

In contemporary American life, the behaviors and rituals that are used to weave illness into everyday living have all but disappeared for many of us. We might drop off a casserole to someone who is sick or visit someone in the hospital, but otherwise the individual goes to the doctor, the pharmacy, and the sickbed alone or perhaps accompanied by a spouse or other family member. The community waits in the wings for the person's recovery and no longer takes an active role in promoting the individual's return to health.

The old healing customs prevented isolation. The family and village would assemble to watch and participate in the shaman's ceremony, and thus patient and caregiver saw their friends and extended family. Now, with the absence of community-centered rituals, with the geographic separation of many extended families, and with the cultural value placed on stoicism, it is too easy for people who are ill or taking care of people who are ill to retreat into their private worlds. We become isolated from our support systems when we most need them.

If you are lucky, you may have a friend or circle of friends who simply won't permit you to isolate yourself. If you are not part of such a circle, find one. Many churches and synagogues have a committee of volunteers who will visit the sick. Some advocacy organizations—such as the American Diabetes Association, the Alzheimer's Association, the National Alliance on Mental Illness, and other disease-specific agencies—host support groups for patients or caregivers.

There are a number of websites that facilitate the creation of a personalized page on which friends and family can sign up to bring meals, help out with errands or chores, or accompany the patient to an appointment or treatment session. You can set up the page yourself or ask a friend to do it for you. Usually people are eager to help, but they don't know what to do. Your friends may be waiting to be told what to do, and they will be happy and relieved when you direct them in how they may help. These websites make it easy to ask for the help you need.

The Psychological Impact of Stress

When the waves close over me, I
dive down to fish for pearls.
—Masha Kaleko

The stress of a loved one's serious illness can exacerbate a pre-existing psychiatric condition in the caregiver or can create a new one. Even the most mentally healthy individuals may develop an adjustment disorder, which is the development of marked anxiety, depression, or behavior change in response to a stressor. Symptoms tend to be disproportionate to the stressor and might cause impairment in daily functioning at home, work, or school.[31] Adjustment disorders are very common in adolescents and adults, and they are treatable with psychotherapy.

If someone has an underlying mental-health problem—such as recurrent major depression, persistent depressive disorder, bipolar disorder, panic disorder, post-traumatic stress disorder, generalized anxiety disorder, a substance-use disorder, or any of dozens of other psychiatric disorders—symptoms may be worsened by stress, including the worry and sleep interruptions that often accompany caring for a medically ill person.

If you are taking medication to manage your mental-health problem, this is the time to pay particular attention to not missing doses. You may need to adjust the dose of your medication to compensate for the added stress. It is wise to meet with the health-care provider monitoring your medication at the earliest

---

31 American Psychiatric Association, *Diagnostic and Statistical Manual of Mental Disorders*, 5th ed. (Washington, DC: American Psychiatric Press, 2013).

sign of a problem rather than wait until you have a full-blown recurrence, which may be harder to treat.

A common error among medical doctors and their patients who are dealing with serious illness is to brush off symptoms of anxiety and depression with the comment, "Of course they're anxious or depressed. I would be, too, if I had MS/AIDS/cancer." The existence of a "good" reason to be depressed or anxious doesn't mean the depression or anxiety should remain untreated.

Many scientific studies have documented that people who have had heart attacks, strokes, or cancer recover better and live longer if their depression is treated. The reasons for this finding are only beginning to be understood, but they include the fact that depression is associated with impairments in the immune system, which is important in fighting cancer. Furthermore, serotonin, one of the neurotransmitters whose imbalance is implicated in depression and anxiety, is also important for good platelet function, which in turn is important in preventing inappropriate clotting, as can occur in strokes and heart attacks. In addition, there is growing evidence that inflammation, which is present in many medical illnesses, is also present in depression.

Major depression impairs sleep, appetite, energy, the ability to think through problems, and the capacity to experience pleasure. Anxiety impairs sleep; the ability to think through problems; the capacity to be in the moment; and body functions including the digestive system, heart rate, and blood pressure. These are vital functions for us all but especially for a caregiver.

Treatment of anxiety and depression will help the caregiver feel emotionally stronger and perform better. Treatment may include antidepressant medication, which also works for anxiety disorders, as well a variety of psychotherapies. Cognitive behavioral therapy (CBT) has been scientifically proven to be as effective as medication for mild to moderate depression and for many of the anxiety disorders. CBT is a short-term therapy (often eight to twelve sessions) that helps the individual identify and correct dysfunctional thoughts and behaviors that perpetuate depression and anxiety.

Interpersonal therapy (IPT) is also effective for major depression. IPT is a brief therapy (often twelve sessions) that helps the individual analyze patterns in his or her relationships and identify how current interpersonal experiences produce emotional symptoms. Other forms of psychotherapy—including psychodynamic therapy, existential therapy, and supportive therapy—may all be especially useful for caregivers. In addition, cardiovascular exercise for at least thirty minutes on most days of the week has been proven to be as effective as medication for relieving mild to moderate depression.

It can make all the difference to your mental health when you work with a therapist to process how you are feeling and to develop strategies and skills to handle the difficulties you encounter in caring for a loved one. Even when you have supportive family members and friends to talk to, a therapeutic alliance with a trained professional can be extremely beneficial. This person can be your lifeline, as you do not have to take care of a clinician's feelings or worry about her reactions the way you might with someone you are close to. The ability to speak candidly and work through some of the troubling emotions you are confronting can make an enormous difference and help you to cope and even thrive during this stressful time of limbo.

Sometimes I feel disembodied from myself. I hear my voice saying, "Advanced lung cancer," and I just can't even believe it's us. I tell the story over and over now almost dispassionately, like I am recounting something that is about someone else. How is this me? How is this us? It all feels like a betrayal that our lives have changed so drastically, so quickly.

If you have doubts about your feelings, it is validating to have a professional tell you that it is normal to feel angry, sad, or anxious. When someone with experience and expertise explains commonly felt physical and emotional symptoms, you may feel comforted that others often react the way you are reacting.

In this day and age, most of us know that seeing a therapist does not mean that something is wrong with you or that you are weak. However, there are some people who still carry stigmatized perceptions (sometimes unconsciously) of what mental-health treatment is about. The old messages of "Pull yourself up by your bootstraps" and "Get over it," which remain a part of our culture, can feel demeaning and diminishing to people who are facing changes and difficulties in their lives. Recognizing when you might benefit from therapy or counseling and allowing yourself to pursue that path can be crucial to your ability to successfully handle your challenges.

If you are uncomfortable with the idea of entering therapy or if you are unable to find a professional you can afford, look for assistance from social workers or chaplains in the clinic in which your loved one is receiving treatment or from another social-services agency or hospice. Most clergy members are also trained to counsel congregants who are in a life crisis or transition.

> Even if you have a trustworthy confidant in your life, consider finding a therapist. A therapist is trained to keep his or her own needs and judgments out of the room so that the focus is entirely on helping you. It is important to find a therapist with whom you feel comfortable, someone you feel understands you and supports you. It is completely acceptable to interview two or three therapists before picking one; some therapists will even offer the initial consultation session for free (although this practice is disappearing).
>
> The category of therapist is quite broad. It includes psychiatrists (who are medical doctors), psychologists (who have a PhD or PsyD), social workers (who have a master's degree in social work), licensed therapists (who must meet the educational requirements, often a master's degree, of the state in which they are licensed), and unlicensed therapists (whose skills and training are variable).

There is an even greater range of types of therapy: from psycho-analysis to short-term group treatment, and everything in be-tween. In addition, some forms of therapy work better for certain kinds of problems than for others. And, of course, some therapists will be covered by your insurance, and others may not be. Where do you start in making a selection?

Your primary-care doctor may be able to suggest a therapist for you, especially if your doctor already has a sense of what the prob-lem is. Also, your primary-care doctor may already refer to thera-pists who are covered by your insurance, if that is important to you. Suggestions from family members or friends who know of good therapists are also a smart place to start. You may not want to see the same person your mother talks to, but that person may be able to give you a list of colleagues he or she respects.

Finding Your Own Self-Care Strategies

> *The purpose of art is washing the*
> *dust of daily life off our souls.*
> —PABLO PICASSO

Artistic endeavors and crafty projects can be great mechanisms for dis-charging stress and exploring self-expression. After Bill's diagnosis, I learned how to knit and enjoyed the mostly mindless, constructive aspect of the craft. It kept my hands and mind busy during hours and hours of waiting in doctors' offices. I also resurrected my dormant ability to play piano, finding it a soothing escape at home. Pulling out my old volume of Chopin waltzes was a way to add beauty to my life, while also allowing me to release some emotional tension. I spent a few weekends painting a bathroom in our house. That project gave me the satisfaction of attaining a tangible result (rich navy walls)—a small piece of my life in which I could actually control the outcome. Over the course of a year, I used the early mornings and late evenings when I was feeling restless to draft a novel.

If you are so inclined, keeping a journal can be a wonderful outlet. It was very therapeutic for me to write down my thoughts and feelings. Often I caught twenty minutes or so between the time my kids went to school and I went to work. I frequently found the pen take on a life of its own, expressing sentiments I wasn't even conscious of feeling. I allowed myself to be free, to not worry about perfect sentence construction. No one else was going to read it (I wasn't anticipating writing this book and using some excerpts), let alone grade it.

> *Writing in this journal helps because I am actually processing my thinking and emotions, as opposed to just lying in a puddle of stagnant thoughts that invoke fear and stress. Instead of merely ruminating, I am telling a story, which makes me feel that I am moving forward.*

As busy as you are, try to carve out some time for creative expression. It can be air and water for your soul.

In addition to getting in touch with your inner artist, many other activities can occupy your time or give you a psychological break. Ideas might include the following: sports (e.g., tennis, running, skiing, going to the gym, bowling), hobbies (e.g., knitting, model building, woodworking), solitary activities (e.g., reading, crossword puzzles, jigsaw puzzles, Sudoku), entertainment (e.g., watching TV, listening to music, playing a video game, having people over), going out (e.g., movies, theater, museum, lunch or coffee with a friend, taking a drive, shopping), household activities (e.g., gardening, baking, decorating, sewing), creative or educational pursuits (e.g., photography, calligraphy, learning a foreign language, writing poems, playing music, painting, dancing), physical and meditative activities (e.g., yoga, exercise, martial arts, hiking, walking the dog), connecting with others (e.g., writing letters, playing games, talking on the phone, joining a club, sex), and soothing comforts (e.g., lighting candles, taking a bath, sunbathing, napping, getting a pedicure).

Self-care can be as simple as sitting quietly and doing deep-breathing exercises or meditating about a favorite place, person, or event in your life.

Even a mental visit to an imaginary destination or having a conversation with a fictional or historical figure who gives you strength can be soothing.

Find activities that feel relaxing or regenerating to you, and be sure to build them into your day.

It is adaptive to carve out time to maintain (or establish) good self-care habits. If you have always used yoga or hikes or facials or attending concerts as ways to relax or nourish yourself, now is not the time to give up these activities. If anything, you want to try to increase your self-care to help sustain your equilibrium while you are stressed. If you never paid much attention to exercise or leisure activities before your loved one became ill, now is the time to start.

This might seem counterintuitive; you might feel that all your spare time must be directed toward taking care of your loved one. Actually, that approach invites burnout. You may recall from high-school physics the law of conservation of energy, which states that energy cannot be created or destroyed; it can only be changed from one form to another.

If you spend energy in an activity, your energy level will be diminished, unless you also tap into an energy source for yourself. It is impossible to continue to expend so much energy on taking care of the physical and emotional needs of someone with a serious illness without finding a way to replenish your reserves. Since you probably won't have as much time to recharge as you devote to expending energy, you want to ensure that your recharge technique is maximally effective and efficient. If you have only one hour, spending it at the mall may not give you as much of a boost as having coffee with a dear friend or exercising with a personal trainer.

If the reality of your situation is that you can't leave your loved one home alone, you can still devote a few minutes of each day to doing some stretches, to meditating, to reading poetry or the newspaper, or to talking to your best friend on the phone. Perhaps you can arrange for a friend, family member, church volunteer, or even a hired professional to stay with your loved one for a few hours once a week, or at least once a month, so you can go for a hike or get a massage or visit a museum—whatever feels most appealing and nourishing to you. (Getting help is discussed later in this chapter.)

Self-care is as important as going to the grocery store. Without it, you risk running out of your supplies of energy, cheerfulness, patience, and empathy.

Managing Caregiver Burnout

> *Do not think that love, in order to be genuine, has to be extraordinary. What we need is to love without getting tired.*
> —Mother Teresa

There are times when the needs of your loved one mesh well with your ability and desire to meet those needs. But what about when they don't? How much should you be expected to do? I have an acquaintance who allows her elderly father to control her by insisting she do everything for him. He will not permit another caregiver in the home, even though they can afford one.

The daughter has a demanding job in a city that is 150 miles from her father, and there are no employment opportunities for her in the small town that her father refuses to leave. Every weekend she makes the long drive to her father's house, prepares his meals for the week, and takes care of everything at his house. Sometimes she goes there midweek for doctors' appointments or emergencies. The daughter has had no social life for many years, as there is no time to date, nurture friendships, or get involved in community activities. Clearly she has allowed this situation to occur, but now she feels completely trapped as her father's medical problems increase.

If you are in a similar predicament, you may find that as time goes on, the situation becomes intractable. You may believe you have lost your ability to extricate yourself from the patterns that you may have been partly responsible for establishing.

Keep in mind that you are a person, too. Your loved one's illness doesn't make him or her more important than you. Think carefully about to what extent you should be expected to sacrifice yourself. A person with a serious illness may understandably be angry, exhausted, or depressed. And those conditions may lead her to be insensitive or ignorant of your needs. Scenarios in which there are high expectations of the caregiver coupled with minimal appreciation for those efforts are prone to a buildup of resentment. It is best to address these perceptions with the ill person or, if she doesn't have the capacity, with a good friend or therapist so that bitter feelings don't fester.

> When someone we love is ill, we want to be kind and compassionate caregivers. At times we may fall short of our ideal. Many factors will play into how often and to what extent we can remain effective caregivers: the degree to which we are rested or tired, the responsibilities demanding our attention, the quality of and degree of conflict in our relationship with the person who is ill, their ability to receive our attention with kindness in return, and many other factors.
>
> Some of these are modifiable, such as making sure we get enough sleep, while others are not under our control, such as the other person's response. If the person you're caring for is suffering from depression or is in physical pain, he or she may not respond with enthusiasm or warmth. While you cannot control that person's response, you can adjust your expectations. Talk to your loved one about what kind of response you would like, and negotiate a response that he or she feels capable of giving even while enduring depression, pain, or malaise.
>
> Much has been written about caregiver burnout. Two general principles mitigate burnout: having a degree of control and

maintaining good self-care. Of course there are many aspects of your loved one's illness over which neither of you have any control and other areas over which your loved one will want to retain control. It is helpful to identify something over which you would like to have a say and that would make you feel that you can influence an element of the events in your loved one's illness.

For example, if poor appetite is a problem for your loved one, you may feel discouraged that she eats little of the food you took time to prepare. It is a good idea, of course, to find out what foods are most palatable, which gives your loved one some control over the menu and helps you to focus your culinary efforts in a successful direction.

In addition, it may help you feel more inspired or motivated if you make some aspect of the meal preparation more pleasant for yourself. You could light a candle next to the stove and put on the music of your choice, turning meal preparation into a little private party. You could establish a pattern that once a week is your night off from the kitchen, and you get to order out. It would be fine for you to order your food from two different restaurants, since you may have a hankering for spicy Indian food, while your loved one's stomach wants nothing more than wonton soup.

Give yourself permission to attend to your own needs for control in these ways. Do not feel guilty about identifying and attending to your own needs. If you are stronger and happier, your loved one benefits, too.

Even the most loving, patient person sometimes gets tired of care-giving. This is not a problem if the person recognizes it, is able to take a restorative break, and has the resources to get some extra help to ward off repeated burnout. Sometimes it is hard to recognize burnout. You may feel irritable or overwhelmed but explain away those feelings as being natural under the circumstances.

You may cry more easily or wake up in the middle of the night with anxiety, but these symptoms, too, are easily brushed aside as understandable reactions to stress. All these feelings are normal, but they can creep insidiously up to a distressing intensity or last longer and longer until they become a pervasive emotional state. Waking up anxious almost every night, crying at the least little thing, snapping with irritability repeatedly during the day, or feeling constantly overwhelmed or out of control are not healthy states of being.

One of the biggest obstacles to recognizing one's burnout is guilt. It may feel unacceptable to acknowledge fatigue, because the person with the illness is worse off than the caregiver. Yet it is unrealistic to expect to meet your loved one's needs without attending to your own needs, too. And as we mentioned before, when you take time to talk to a friend or therapist, eat well, exercise, or relax with a good book, you replenish yourself for the continued tasks of caregiving. These are not selfish luxuries; they are critical, self-sustaining activities, like putting gas in the tank and air in the tires, without which you will have a hard time continuing on your journey.

Getting Help and Taking Breaks

No act of kindness, no matter how small, is ever wasted.
—AESOP

Part of caring for your loved one includes arranging time when you aren't interacting with him or her. It is important to give yourself permission to take breaks, since it only makes things worse if you are worn down and beleaguered. Even if your loved one resists your stealing respites here or there, remember to attend to your own susceptibility to fatigue and stress.

When adults travel with children, they are instructed by the flight attendant that in the event of an emergency, they should put on their own oxygen masks before assisting others. They then can take care of the children with their full capacity. If instead the adult passes out while attending first to the children, everyone is in trouble. It is like that with supporting a friend or family member with an illness. Attending only to the patient's needs while ignoring your own will be detrimental to all.

If your loved one is a spouse or partner who participated in household work, you may find yourself in a position in which you are suddenly doing twice as much as you used to, in and out of the home. This can exacerbate your sense of being overwhelmed and stressed.

> *This morning I came outside, and Bill hadn't put out the trash. Why did that make me so sad? That he forgot? That he didn't feel up to it? That one of these days, months, years, I may be the only one to do it? It's so hard that something as small as that can make me feel so devastated just because of all of its implications.*

One of the first chores that Bill had to give up was shoveling the snow. He just did not have the lung capacity to hoist heavy loads out in the cold. Shoveling had been an enjoyable task for him, as he had valued the combination of a productive activity, fresh air, and an extra workout all in one. For me, it was an unpleasant chore. In all our years of marriage, I had almost never shoveled the walks and driveway. One day after his diagnosis, when I was outside lifting the shovel after a particularly massive snowfall, I found tears streaming down my face.

It wasn't that I felt sorry for myself because I had to shovel the walk, but instead I felt heartbroken for both of us, because we were too young to be in the position where Bill was losing such simple capabilities. Although he was still active and going to work, limitations were starting to slowly creep into his life. Was this just the beginning of the new reality that would slowly chip away at our comfortable routines and lifestyle? It seemed that we were starting on a new trajectory toward weakness and infirmity, a realization that filled me with sorrow.

At the same time, illness can cause family members to adapt to new roles and responsibilities. An elderly man we knew ended up in a caregiving role for his wife, who gradually lost her functionality due to a progressive neurological illness. Almost sixty years into their marriage, I don't think he had actually been all the way into the kitchen past the table where his wife had always served him his meals. Gradually he learned to make coffee, run and empty the dishwasher, and fix some easy items at the stove.

As we mentioned in chapter 3, the rest of your life doesn't stop when crisis hits, although it can feel like it has or, at the very least, should. Most everything that you were doing before will still need to get done after the diagnosis. And then some.

Carefully consider what you must do, what you can let go, and what you might be able to delegate. If you can afford it, hire someone to clean your house, mow your lawn, or perform other household chores. If hired help isn't financially realistic, do you have friends or neighbors you can ask to pitch in? Not everything can be handled personally by you, nor does it need to be. When you chart out your to-do list, try to limit the items you absolutely insist stay in your purview. Spare yourself when you have the opportunity and a willing volunteer or paid worker to give you a hand.

> *Today when Bill's friends came over to clean out the garage, I felt so touched that these guys came up with such a useful, thoughtful gift. But it is awkward to me for them to be doing this for us. I'm comfortable being the giver, not being on the receiving end.*

The bottom line is you cannot do everything yourself—even if you want to. Let people in. Look to your family and friends for support in ways in which you all feel comfortable, and think of specific things that will be helpful and ease your burden.

Here are some ideas: Would you be able to take my cat to the vet? Could you sit with our loved one during chemo next Friday? Are you available to pick up my kids from school tomorrow when we are at a doctor's appointment? Might you help me write thank-you notes for food and gifts? Do you think you could call the insurance company and find out why they didn't cover this procedure? Would you mind taking my brother-in-law to the airport on Sunday? If they can do it, your friends will usually appreciate getting a specific assignment.

Some people shrink away from help offered by others. They want to feel "normal" as much as possible. For example, my children clearly felt awkward when friends brought us meals and greatly preferred the comfort and routine of my cooking. Since making dinner is a pleasant activity for me, I continued for the most part to fix our meals, keeping them simple and familiar.

> Sometimes offers of help can feel intrusive. If your sister-in-law from out of town wants to come for an extended visit to help out, but you don't get along well with her, you may need to negotiate a compromise. Ask her what she has in mind, and then establish parameters for the visit ahead of time.

> If she offers to take the children to school every morning, but that's an important part of your daily routine that you don't want to give away, tell her that what would really help would be for her to walk the family dog each morning while you take the kids to school (for example). Ask her for how long and where she plans to stay. Hosting a three-week guest in your home may not feel helpful to you. But if she stays in a nearby inn, offers to pitch in with the laundry and housekeeping, and watches the kids on Saturday nights so that you can go out on a date with your spouse, you may discover a new appreciation for your sister-in-law.

> Don't be afraid to check out all her expectations so that they can be adjusted. Does she plan to join you for every meal? If she's staying in your house, does she expect you to make breakfast for her, like you do for your kids? If you need more privacy, how will you broach the subject? If these topics have been introduced ahead of time, it may be easier to raise them again without bruising each other's feelings. On the other hand, if you and your sister-in-law

cannot have this kind of negotiation, then it may be better to politely decline her visit.

In addition to some of your household chores, if your loved one needs quite a bit of care, look for ways of hiring help or finding available volunteer services. These may include Meals on Wheels, a companion or sitter for a person with dementia, or out-of-home day care. Various health-care agencies and nonprofit organizations provide professionals or lay volunteers who will come to your house to help with medications, exercises, bathing, and getting dressed; to provide physical, occupational, or mental-health therapy; or to conduct skilled nursing.

Finding the right caregivers can be difficult and an ongoing process. I recently asked a relative whether she had found stable care for her mother. She replied, "She's shown up every day since Monday." (It was Wednesday.)

This is a good time to use word-of-mouth sources for accessing and assessing competent, reliable care. Some people prefer to use an agency; others hire caregivers directly. In either case, close oversight is a must. I have a friend who was able to secure excellent care for her father by finding nurses from the hospital who were interested in moonlighting. If you cannot afford to hire a private caregiver, contact human- or family-service agencies to see if there are free or low-cost programs you might access.

Taking care of someone with a serious illness or disability is very demanding work, physically and emotionally. Make sure the caregivers you have hired have adequate breaks and aren't working unreasonably long shifts. And as is sometimes the case, you may need to intervene if the ill person is disrespectful or abusive to the caregiver. It is not uncommon for people who are sick to take out their anger or frustration on someone whom they perceive to be subordinate. Kindness and consideration go a long way to holding on to good care providers and making them feel appreciated.

If Your Relationship Is Difficult or Strained

We must let go of the life we have planned, so
as to accept the one that is waiting for us.
—JOSEPH CAMPBELL

In *Social Intelligence: The New Science of Human Relationships*, Daniel Goleman discusses the emotional economy and the ways in which our inner gains and losses can affect our interactions with other people. Both negative and positive emotions can be contagious; we can catch certain feelings from one another. Spending a lot of time with a person who is miserable can bring us down, too. As we care for someone, Goleman explains, we attune ourselves to his or her inner state. That person's emotions penetrate us. If those feelings are unwanted or destructive, we need to find a way to alter their impact. In the same way, *our* negative emotions can have a toxic effect on others. If we are in a situation in which we are producing reciprocal negativity, we can end up making a difficult time much worse.[32]

How do you, as the caregiver, get what you need? Or how do you cope and find peace if you don't get what you want? Through the suggestions in this section of the book, look for what works for you, whether it is engaging a therapist or close confidant, finding a support group or meaningful readings, or some of the many suggested self-care techniques. Try to recognize that a person who is ill often feels powerless, so when he is controlling or takes his caregiver for granted, it may only be his attempt to find a small vestige of power over his life.

Even in a healthy, loving relationship, illness can change the dynamics of our interactions. I often found myself protecting Bill from my anxieties about his prognosis, just as he had a tendency to protect me by not fully disclosing how he was feeling. It was clear to me that in these ways we weren't being as honest with each other as we had been throughout our relationship, which was a new and undesired consequence of the illness.

---

32 Daniel Goleman, *Social Intelligence: The New Science of Human Relationships* (New York: Bantam, 2006).

I know of some cases in which the situation became so untenable that difficult choices had to be made. I have a work colleague whose wife suffered from severe mental illness that made it impossible for their family to function in a healthy way. After many years of giving his absolute best effort to support his wife, my colleague decided that the ramifications of the disease were taking too big of a toll on him and their young son. The wife had long been unable to work and often required inpatient psychiatric treatment or in-home care.

Not only were her needs draining the family's economic resources, but also her emotional outbursts and rage were abusive and not successfully mitigated by therapy or medications. The husband could not continue to sacrifice his and his child's welfare, as their lives had truly become a living nightmare. He knew that none of this was his wife's fault, but still he needed to plan for his son's education, their mortgage, and other expenses. With such a huge chunk of his income going to maintain his wife's treatment and care, he felt forced to leave her so that she could access public services and also remove his son from the harmful environment.

Another way conflict can arise is when the loved one chooses not to adhere to medical advice. A friend recently told me that her neighbor is choosing not to follow the recommended treatment for his neurological illness. Although several promising treatments are available, he does not want to pursue them. Meanwhile, his wife is feeling frustrated and resentful that her husband will not try to lessen the symptoms and severity of his illness. It compounds the burden the wife is already feeling when she believes her spouse is not doing his part to lessen the impact this illness is having on their lives and the pressure she feels to make significant sacrifices.

Deciding what to do in these troubling circumstances depends on many factors, including financial and emotional resources. This is a time to discuss options with professionals, such as your therapist, an attorney, a clinic social worker, or private or public human-services organizations.

CHAPTER 8
Making Decisions

I n this chapter, we address ways of interacting with the health-care system, including gathering information, making care decisions, and communicating with other involved people. Integral considerations in this aspect of the process are styles of medical decision-making, the utility of second opinions, how to approach ambiguous information, and speaking up as a patient advocate.

Defining Roles

> *Determine the thing that can and shall be*
> *done, and then we shall find the way.*
> —Abraham Lincoln

When your loved one is sick or disabled, your role is not only demanding and emotional but also complex and multifaceted. You may need to be advocate, caregiver, cheerleader, researcher, and therapist all at once. The first thing to do is determine what your loved one needs and what you are capable of providing. Respect your limitations. For example, if you have back trouble, you cannot be in a position where you must lift someone who is weak. If you have a hard time grasping medical information, you should not be the only one receiving it. Have a conversation with the person who is ill and with other family members to negotiate your respective roles.

Judging the competence of your loved one to make decisions is an ongoing task, since mental and emotional function may change over time. Watch for cognitive impairment or depression, which may accompany or result from the underlying illness. Your loved one may be competent for some things but not for others. For example, a person with moderate dementia may not be mentally competent to process new information in order to make thoughtful decisions about her treatment, while she is still able to establish with her family her clear preferences about the care of household and personal needs.

Some people with illnesses prefer to do as little as possible in presiding over their own cases, while others want complete independence in assessing and choosing the course of treatment. We had a friend with cancer who spent a huge amount of his time on his laptop poring over any available information about his diagnosis, while another preferred to let her husband do this job and wanted to confront her cancer only when she was sitting in the oncologist's office.

A relative with particular expertise (especially one who is a doctor) may engender or expect deference from the rest of the family. But sometimes friends and family members with medical backgrounds do not want to be pulled into this role, especially if the illness or disability is far afield from their expertise. When this is the case, it may be appropriate to ask such people to explain technical medical terms or conditions to you but not to give you their medical advice. These friends may also be willing to check out the credentials of a particular physician or the reputation of a treatment facility for you.

It may be helpful and healthy to have authority divided up, giving people different responsibilities. The husband of a woman with an illness may choose to continue making financial decisions while deferring to his daughter to help her mother make medical decisions. Coming to familial or group consensus about who is in charge of what and reevaluating these decisions as needed can help to mitigate strife, as limbo can be exhausting and tense for everyone.

Sometimes a family member who undertakes the brunt of the responsibility for the person with the illness feels judged or criticized by other family members for his decisions, which exacerbates his stress. For example, if a sibling who is choosing a more peripheral role in the care of her mother decides to criticize her brother for hiring outside caregivers, then he may decide to ask his sister to step up to the plate. Sometimes family members argue over the impact their loved one's care might have on their ultimate inheritance. The strain of illness can reveal motives that may be self-serving and not in the best interest of the person who is sick. A family conference may be necessary to come to consensus on important issues of care and paying for it.

Family relationships can become strained or even break down in cases where there is a conflict or competition over who is in charge. While the capacity and wishes of the person with the illness are the most important considerations, in some situations, that person's vulnerability or incompetence will cause a dominating personality to step in, and that person's approach may or may not be congruent with the other family members or the stated wishes of the loved one.

In a family I knew, the elderly father had a second recurrence of his cancer. Although he had valiantly battled the disease during the first two go-rounds, he decided he didn't have the energy or the will to do it again. Rather than face the grueling treatment and its likely side effects, he chose to refuse treatment and let nature take its course. While one of his children was immediately supportive of this decision, the other two could not accept the idea that their father was willing to let the illness take him without a fight. This difference of opinion caused friction in the family, which was not resolved until they all had to concur that the father was of sound mind and that they had no choice but to get on board with his decision. I remember thinking about how much more complicated it might have been had there been a disagreement about the father's competence to make this decision.

The powerful emotions that surface when a family member is ill may cause strains and estrangements that can last well beyond the health crisis. I have known families who have never recovered from the stresses that arose during a loved one's illness. It can be helpful to access your highest reserves of compassion and self-compassion to maneuver sensitive family roles and expectations.

> When a patient is not in agreement with his or her physician about the treatment plan or when a family member is not in agreement with a patient about a course of action, the tension may be very uncomfortable. In many cases, if the people who are in disagreement can stay engaged in a dialogue, resolution will come. On the other hand, if people get entrenched in their positions, the disagreement becomes polarized, an obstacle to negotiation or compromise.

> Be patient with ambiguity and disagreement. It is useful to remind yourself that life is a process, not an outcome. At various stages of the process, you may face uncertainty, ambiguity, or conflict, all of which may cause distress.

Finding the Right Doctor

Our main business is not to see what lies dimly in
the distance but to do what lies clearly at hand.
—Thomas Carlyle

When the diagnosis is initially made, the first task may be figuring out where to go for treatment. This decision may be dependent on whether you live in a big city with specialists in the field or in a small town without the medical resources you need. This is a time to consult with any contacts whom you think might be helpful. Your primary-care doctor should be able to give you appropriate referrals, but do not hesitate to also ask friends or family members to help guide you. If your loved one is going to need ongoing, long-term treatment, it is obviously preferable to find care in your community, where the rest of your life is located, but that is not always possible.

If there is more than one good option, check them out. The first oncologist we interviewed was quite personable and seemed perfectly knowledgeable and competent. But when several people urged us to see another doctor, we decided after both visits that the second one was a better choice. We hesitated to call the first doctor to decline his offer of care after he had spent two hours consulting with us, but we had to remind ourselves that our only consideration was accessing the best care possible. We knew that this decision could (and I believe did) make a big difference in the treatment Bill received.

I have learned over the years that there is a wide range of attitudes about the act of seeking a second opinion. In medical training, we are taught to view second opinions as a good idea, a way to corroborate one's decision-making or to elicit helpful suggestions from a respected colleague.

It was at first confusing to me that my patients would seem hurt or embarrassed if I raised the topic of a second opinion. If I suggest a second opinion, some patients think I'm trying to get rid of them by disguising a transfer of care as a consultation. Other patients get defensive on my behalf, rushing to reassure me that they have confidence in my care, as if asking for a second opinion is an admission of incompetence. Similarly, if the patient asks for a second opinion, it is often couched in apology: "I think you're terrific, but my parents/spouse/friends think I should see someone their own doctor knows."

For me, a second opinion is a useful resource, especially if I know that the doctor providing the second opinion has particular expertise in the problem in question. I am almost always happy to support a patient's request for a second opinion. The only exception is when the patient chooses the consulting physician's name from a long list provided by their insurance company, without regard for the provider's expertise. If you're going to go to the trouble of getting a second opinion, it probably makes sense to see an expert, even if it costs more.

Being a Good Consumer

The best way out is always through.
—ROBERT FROST

One lesson that I need to metabolize is that this whole treatment course is going to be evolving and changing as we go along. Rather than thinking, "OK we have 12 weeks of this treatment and then one year of that one," we have to be in the mental framework of "We are doing this treatment for 3 weeks, and we'll see how it goes."

As much as I tried to be what they call a "good consumer" in this process, I often felt insecure, because without a strong scientific background, I just couldn't understand all the medical information that confronted us. Plus, since much of the data were so upsetting, this information exacerbated feelings of anxiety and helplessness. This was especially true of the numbers that turned Bill into a cold statistic. As we got into the area of experimental treatments and clinical trials, we became even more overwhelmed. In one sitting, we found 199 trials nationally on Bill's specific type of cancer. Almost all the science in these descriptions was completely over our heads.

The Internet can be a mixed blessing. With a wealth of information now available at the click of a mouse, we consumers have the opportunity to be much better informed and prepared. It is remarkable how much you can learn from one session in front of your computer. Stories of hope may provide just the inspiration you need to get through your day. Reports of a new drug therapy may arm you with important questions for the doctor. But remember, the Internet can also be a repository of misinformation and false hope. At best, erroneous or misunderstood information can distract you, and at worst, it can leave you devastated.

Shortly into our journey, we were very encouraged by a website allegedly written by a woman with Bill's exact diagnosis who had a surgery that completely eliminated her cancer. When we excitedly reported this to Bill's doctor, an internationally known oncologist in his field, he said the surgery this woman described was utterly impossible.

There are many so-called cures offered up on the Internet, in magazines, and by word of mouth: herbal remedies, treatments available only in other countries, and expensive therapies not based on any evidence. Even if a prospect isn't an out-and-out scam, you should always approach obscure remedies with skepticism. You have to wonder why your mainstream physician who reads all the current medical journals has not heard of a supposed cure that you find on a random website. Stick with reputable sources, such as leading associations dedicated to the relevant illness, major medical institutions, or governmental research centers.

You may find, as we did, that it is necessary to enlist some help in this area. Is there someone in your life who can be your researcher and interpreter? It may be a relative or friend who is already providing support to you, or it might be a person who has completely different skills from the nurturing confidant at your side. If at all possible, try to find someone who is smart, conscientious, and reliable, a person who is computer savvy and willing to read and sift through information for you. Ideally he or she will glean what you need to know (omitting horrifying statistics if you so request) and, most importantly, help you frame questions for the doctor.

Even though I often surprised myself at how much I could handle, reading about Bill's illness was not something I ever mastered. Browsing relevant websites or bookstore shelves always caused my stomach to churn, my heart to race, and my head to throb. Panic would set in as I pondered grim prognoses, potential complications, or dwindling prospects for treatment. Neither Bill nor I found it beneficial to plow through facts and figures that were usually discouraging. At the same time, there were things we needed to know: treatments to ask about, information that would equip us to make the most of his doctor's appointments.

We were fortunate that my sister and my mother willingly and capably took on this role, preparing a list of questions before each appointment based on Bill's current symptoms and research they did on new developments in treatment. Neither of them had a medical background, but they quickly educated themselves enough to provide us the information we would need to perform well in this decision-making capacity. It helped shield us from the giant onslaught of available information, some of which was disconcerting or questionable, leaving us adequately prepared and competent when we had our precious time with the doctor.

Given that neither Bill nor I had a background in medicine, when we would meet with the doctor, what we desperately wanted was for him to tell us what to do. While we might not have come out and said, "You decide," we would try every possible way to get him to tell us what he thought was best. The problem was that we were traveling in new territories where solid evidence was not yet available.

One time we were at one of the forks in the road, and the treatment options were numerous, while their relative merits were unclear. Our doctor sat us down and said (essentially), "You can do A or B or A and B together or C alone or with D or A and C together. Also there is E, which you can do alone or combined with F."

Our obvious response was, "What do *you* think we should do?"

He answered that all these treatments had shown "*some* efficacy in *some* people," but head-to-head trials on these medications had not yet been completed. How could we choose? We would try to trap our doctor by saying, "If Bill were your family member, what would you do?" He wouldn't bite and instead repeated, "You can do A or B or A and B together…"

It is natural to wish that someone with superior knowledge and experience will guide us down the right course and spare us from making difficult choices ourselves. However, we have to learn to accept that in a world of ever-changing options and inconclusive data, we often find ourselves making major decisions based on not much more than an educated guess.

> Gone are the days of the paternalistic doctor who makes all the decisions for the passive and conciliatory patient. Most doctors in practice today have been trained in a model of collaborative decision-making, in which the doctor's job is to educate the patient about the illness and its treatments and the patient's job is

to participate in deciding on the treatment plan based on that information.

In my practice, most patients respond enthusiastically to this approach. I like it when people bring in their lists of symptoms, side effects, and questions, because it helps me know that I'm addressing all their concerns. It shows me that the patient is taking an active role in his or her treatment, working at least as hard as I am on our mutual goal of treating the illness. Only rarely does someone say to me after I've presented treatment options, "You're the doctor. You decide."

When my patient wants me to decide, and there isn't a scientific basis to say that one option is superior to another, I use my intuition to choose the treatment plan. But who's to say that my intuition is better than my patient's?

Staying Astute, Vigilant, and Assertive

Luck is when opportunity meets preparation.
—ROBERT EVANS

Because it is easy to get overwhelmed in the physician's office, I began the practice of starting a list several days before each appointment with all the questions I could think of for the doctor. As I mentioned previously, I had help with this task so that our appointments could be as thorough as possible. I found that if I didn't have things written down, I might forget to ask something and then kick myself, because we would then have to postpone that issue for the next appointment or endure the angst of waiting for a return phone call, which invariably came from a busy nurse who did not have personal knowledge of Bill's case.

In addition, it became routine for me to take notes during the appointments, because I often had trouble accurately remembering what was said when I tried to recall or explain certain discussions later. This also tamed my tendency to remember only the most negative, pessimistic comments and to shortchange those that were more encouraging.

To make well-reasoned decisions, we needed to absorb and process complicated medical information. After a couple of visits, Bill's oncologist must have realized that, despite the fact that we appeared intelligent and capable, we were relying on our poor recollections of ninth-grade biology to follow what he was saying. Fortunately, this doctor was detailed with his explanations—even to the point of drawing pictures for us—but still I always felt uncomfortable about my relatively shallow level of understanding and had to learn not to be shy about asking him to repeat information I didn't understand. Since we were facing some of the most critical decisions in our lives, this was not a time to politely feign that I was grasping an explanation, the way I might with my trusted car mechanic.

This was also not a time for us to downplay side effects or other negative aspects of Bill's treatment. The doctor needed this information in order to make sound treatment decisions, as often there were ways to handle adverse reactions while continuing with the course of treatment.

Recently, as I was writing this section, I had an interesting conversation with a psychiatrist friend, who shared his observation about the piercing alertness that patients seem to have when they watch and listen to their doctors. This is something I noticed in myself as I vigilantly scrutinized Bill's oncologist for any facial expressions or gestures that might betray his verbal assertions or reveal his true thoughts. I studied him carefully and treated every word he said as if it were the gospel and every nonverbal cue as highly revelatory.

If he was friendly, I was elated. If he was cold, I was distraught. I read his mannerisms and mood as harbingers of Bill's future. The power he unwittingly wielded over my state of mind just by stepping into the examination room was palpable. If this sounds familiar, my advice is that you keep in mind that doctors are people, too. They have good days and bad days that actually have nothing to do with you and your loved one. They have their own personal and professional burdens that may affect their interactions with their patients, so it is important not to place too much significance on every shrug, sigh, or raising of the brow.

We know from research on human intelligence that we organize and process information according to schemas. A schema is a plan or model based on past experience that we use to understand present experience and predict future outcomes. For example, you may have a schema that helps you anticipate how an initial meeting with a new doctor will go. Your schema is colored by past encounters with doctors and by your general assumptions and attitudes about yourself and the world.

If you have had good experiences with medical providers and generally experience yourself as an effective communicator, your schema for the initial meeting may include an expectation of being heard, eagerness to discuss the problem with the doctor, and anticipation of learning about the treatment choices available to you.

If, on the other hand, you have had negative encounters with medical providers, or if you believe you are not important or intelligent enough to deserve the doctor's time and attention, your schema for a meeting with a new doctor may include anticipation of feeling intimidated, rushed, or confused. Regardless of what actually happens in the meeting with the doctor, your schema will color your thoughts and behaviors and likely will influence the course of the meeting.

Most of the time, our schemas are preconscious; that is, they are not in the front of our awareness, and they operate behind the scenes. It is helpful to be conscious of our schemas so that we can be mindful of their influence. It is possible to amend a maladaptive schema to change your experience in the world.

For example, if you have a distorted schema about initial visits with doctors, such as a belief that doctors never listen to patients, you may feel there's little point in trying to communicate your concerns to the doctor, in which case the doctor won't know to address those concerns, reaffirming your belief that doctors are unresponsive. If you amend your schema to include the possibility that a doctor will have the time and interest to listen to your concerns, you are more likely to speak up, increasing your chances of being heard and of having your concerns addressed.

Today's hospitals and medical clinics are high-pressure, demanding places where many people in different situations vie for the attention of the staff, especially the doctors. In this fast-paced environment, we are forced to make every minute count when we finally have the floor. While preparation is key to maximizing the effectiveness of our interactions with medical personnel, assertiveness is crucial, too. It is best to refrain from being obnoxiously pushy, but in most cases, the proverbial squeaky wheels prevail.

The role we play in being attentive can contribute immensely to effective care and prevent mistakes from occurring. Many people can recite stories of times when they averted a potential disaster by providing a piece of medical history or stopping a near medication error. This is not a criticism of nurses or physicians but just a reality of the often-chaotic circumstances of practice, especially in emergency rooms, where many of us, unfortunately, become repeat customers.

Several years ago, a friend of mine suffered an injury that left her in severe, chronic pain requiring a series of surgeries. Throughout her multiple hospitalizations, she was treated by various physicians on duty, usually a different one every day. Her devoted husband, retired from his job, was always by her side. He was a repository of information about his wife's history, including crucial information about medications that had previously caused an adverse reaction or procedures that had already proven ineffective. While I presume that most of this information was in her chart, I imagine that medical record must have been quite thick after years of treatments in different venues, and critical data could be overlooked in the hurried doctors' visits to her room. My friend lamented that the only thing consistent about her care throughout the ordeal was her husband, a graphic artist with no medical background.

Although it can be intimidating and disheartening to be thrust into the role of medical advocate, you may be in a position where this is the reality. The more you know the big picture and your loved one's medical history, the better care he or she will receive. It can be prudent to keep a notebook with the names of all current medications and their doses, as well as a history of past medications and procedures and other treating physicians' names and contact information, so that you are prepared to answer questions and intervene if necessary.

CHAPTER 9
Toward Inner Peace

This chapter takes a philosophical and spiritual view of adaptation. We can relieve our suffering and achieve a deep acceptance of our new reality by releasing previous expectations. Although people have diverse experiences of faith, it is a useful source of hope and resilience in all its many forms. As we integrate the new perspectives we have gained through the process of adapting to our loved one's illness, we may find ourselves subtly yet profoundly changed. A new awareness of inner peace or joy may emerge.

Serenity, Surrender, and Acceptance

> *In letting go, we release our mental pictures of how things*
> *should turn out and accept what the universe brings us.*
> *We accept that we really don't know how things should be.*
> —ELISABETH KÜBLER-ROSS AND DAVID KESSLER

Today I had lunch with S, and we talked about looking for the opportunities in challenging times. She talked about getting to a place where you are no longer resisting what is happening. It is the idea of surrender. When you truly realize you don't have control, you give up resistance and just live your life. Since control is just an illusion, my state of mind won't affect the outcome of Bill's treatment. His future will be what it will be, independent of whether I am positive or negative about it.

Often, when we are unhappy or disappointed with the circumstances of our lives, we find ourselves wishing things were different. We know rationally that our yearnings are not going to change anything, but still we hold on to them. A few months after Bill's diagnosis, I had dinner with the mother of a boy on my son's baseball team. She was in a situation similar to mine and spent a long time telling me how she just wanted things to be the way they used to be and longed so much for those days when her husband didn't have cancer.

When I responded that returning to that time simply wasn't a choice, she gave me an anguished look, as though I were insensitively throwing water on the burning embers of her past. Even though her husband's illness was quite advanced, she was clearly not willing or able to accept the situation she was in. Her mother-in-law was in town taking care of her husband and kids while she withdrew, desperately clinging to a scenario that was sadly gone.

Somehow we have to get to a place where we are at peace with our situation, rather than dwell in a pretend alternate universe where our loved one is well. We must find serenity in our real lives, limbo and all.

When I was working through some of these ideas about peace and serenity, my sister, who is a hospice chaplain, referred me to a relevant article that she has used in her interactions with patients and families. In the article "'Are You at Peace?': One Item to Probe Spiritual Concerns at the End of Life,"

Steinhauser discusses how in the case of illness, a sense of peacefulness may emerge from different contexts.

From a *biomedical* standpoint, the feeling of being at peace may come from making a clear decision about treatment or managing pain. A *psychosocial* sense of peace may stem from resolving a conflict with a loved one or within oneself. A *spiritual* coming to peace may be based in finding meaning in life, especially as it relates to the illness. Therefore, "Resolution within the biomedical, psycho-social or spiritual domains of patients' experiences often preceded the subjective experience of peacefulness."[33] The same can be true for the caregiver, as we incorporate these different sectors of our own lives in our quest to experience a state of being at peace.

In some of the reading I did early in this journey, I came across the Buddhist concept of surrender. At first I rejected that term, because I felt that it implied defeat, giving up. Bill and I were determined to fight this disease with all our might. But gradually I came to understand that "surrender" can be viewed in a positive way: as acceptance. We surrender to the reality that certain events will just be out of our control, no matter how hard we work or wish to have them resolve in our favor. When we surrender, we give up our resistance and become fully present to live our lives.

I know someone who was dealt a series of health complications in succession. She went from being a busy, successful professional to living a life full of pain and medical setbacks. She would say, "I don't understand this. I've been a good person my whole life. I'm ethical and moral. I don't deserve what has happened to me. There are terrible people out there who are unfaithful, mean, and corrupt. So why did this happen to me? It doesn't make any sense."

In my view, this woman compounded her pain by her childlike perspective of reward and punishment. If you are good, good things will happen. If you are bad, bad things will happen. Even though at a practical level, we all understand that life is not fair, I think many people subconsciously function with this black-and-white mind-set about the universe.

We all hold our own perspectives on the role of a higher power, and these beliefs are personal and may be extremely powerful. In my case, I gave this friend my opinion that her medical problems were not meted out but instead just happened. They were not the by-products of some supernatural umpire making an unfair call. She seemed unable to hear this, because her sense of justice in life was so ingrained in her psyche. Instead she would turn around

---

33   Karen E. Steinhauser, "'Are You at Peace?': One Item to Probe Spiritual Concerns at the End of Life," *Arch Intern Med Archives of Internal Medicine* 166, no. 1 (2006): 101.

and say the same things about my situation: "This is so unfair to Bill, you, and the children. Bill is such a decent human being. He doesn't deserve this."

No one "deserves" to develop cancer or ALS or multiple sclerosis or bipolar illness. No one "deserves" to spend years fighting one illness after another. I believe we need to surrender to the idea that we lack control over these circumstances. Constantly engaging in this type of psychological struggle, like my friend, takes focus away from where it is needed. We must think hard before we spend our precious energy on trying to resist circumstances that can't be resisted.

We all employ strategies to adjust to circumstances that overwhelm us, but as existential theorist Irvin Yalom expresses, when our healthy mechanisms break down, we may go to "extreme measures" to protect ourselves. Two defenses that can surface are a "deep irrational belief in our own specialness" and a "belief in the existence of a personal omnipotent intercessor." In the former case, we think we are too exceptional for natural laws to apply to us, while in the latter, we wait to be rescued by a benevolent power. While these beliefs may be adaptive to a certain point, they also can lead us to the unhealthy place of psychopathology.[34]

> While writing this section, we became curious about the phonetic similarity of the words serene and surrender. Although they sound similar, they are actually from vastly different roots. Serene has its origin in the Latin serenus (of the clear sky). Surrender is from the Latin reddere, which led to the French rendre (to give back) and se rendre (to give oneself up).[35] In Buddhist philosophy, surrender may lead to serenity, in the sense that when we stop fighting against our pain, we may come to peace with it. Similarly, in psychotherapy, when people accept or give themselves up to the feelings that underlie their symptoms, they will achieve a mental clarity about the feelings that often allows the symptoms to clear up.

---

34 Irvin D. Yalom, *Existential Psychotherapy* (New York: Basic Books, 1980).

35 Joseph Shipley, *Dictionary of Word Origins* (New York: Philosophical Library, 1945), 319, 345, and 393.

There may be times when you become so overwhelmed with your life that you can think only, *I can't believe this. I can't believe this is happening.* You might feel so stuck in the mire of your pain that you begin to think it will never end. It can be extremely difficult to accept or adapt to the new construct that is now your reality. There were times when I felt like a refugee from my own (prediagnosis) life, where I had been so comfortable and content, now facing the incessant hardship of my disbelief and sadness. While I knew rationally that I needed to incorporate this uninvited paradigm into my psyche, it was a constant mental battle. And battles, I have found, are fatiguing and demoralizing.

It can be helpful to imagine yourself leaving the war zone. Step off of the battlefield, and let go of trying to win. When you stop engaging in the fight, you are released to pay attention to the things that truly matter to you.

> Marsha Linehan, a psychologist who developed dialectical-behavior therapy, introduced the term "radical acceptance." Derived from both Eastern and Western religious beliefs, radical acceptance is based on the idea that acceptance is the way to turn intolerable suffering into bearable suffering. She calls it "radical" because the acceptance must be complete and deep, not merely lip service. Radical acceptance implies a complete letting go of fighting against the pain in your reality.
>
> Linehan posits that suffering is the combination of pain and nonacceptance of the pain. It is impossible to live with your pain if you refuse to accept it as part of your reality. The nonacceptance interferes with the ability to see, assess, and adapt to your pain. Acceptance is not resignation. Rather, acceptance opens up the possibility for change. Acceptance requires an inner commitment to turn toward reality, which then permits a new experience of your reality.[36]

---

36 Marsha M. Linehan, *Skills Training Manual for Treating Borderline Personality Disorder* (New York: Guilford Press, 1993).

One of my HIV-positive patients, a woman with severe neuropathy pain who was using such high doses of pain medication to try to obliterate the pain that she was sometimes too sedated to get out of bed, applied the concept of radical acceptance with great results. Her pain interfered with her ability to work or care for her children, and it led her physicians to wonder if she was a drug addict. Despite the high doses of narcotics, she still experienced severe pain.

Once she came to the realization that her pain was a permanent part of her life and that she would always feel it, she was able to decide to set the pain aside and get on with the rest of her life. She still felt the pain; it was too strong to ignore. But having accepted that it would be her constant companion, the woman was able to turn her focus to other aspects of her life. Her use of narcotics went down; her alertness and energy went up; and her depression improved, because she felt less victimized by the pain.

Nonattachment

> *You cannot step into the same river twice.*
> —HERACLITUS

There is a Buddhist idea that to live fully in the present, you have to get less invested in specific outcomes, that you can appreciate what you have right now rather than making your happiness contingent on something else—I would be happy "if." I can't live my life under the constant influence of contingencies: "I would be happy if the doctor tells us the medicine is working; I would be happy if he gets better." I have to train myself to appreciate the present with no strings attached, with no contingencies weighing in.

When I first came across readings based on Buddhist philosophy, I was troubled by what I understood to be an instruction to detach from life so that you are essentially neutral toward or immune from all the complications and grief that result from attachments to people and events. My interpretation was that by cultivating a lack of attachment, you are protected from potential sorrow. I could not understand why it would be beneficial to separate psychologically from the very people and events that give your life meaning.

As I read more and continued to reflect on these teachings, I came to realize that I'd misunderstood attachment in this context. Instead, the idea is that when we view everything as outside ourselves and as potential sources of happiness or misery, then we allow our state of mind to be contingent on those other things. If we become too attached to our expectations and dreams for the future, we can feel disillusioned or even devastated if our life takes a different turn than we anticipated. When our state of inner peace is independent of external factors, only then can we truly experience life in the present.

At this point in my life, I am trying to internalize the realization that contentment and fulfillment are not found outside of us. Of course we care deeply about our loved ones. Of course we are devastated when tragic events occur. But if there is one thing I have learned in the past years, it is that joy and peace are found within. Most of my life, I was very much invested in things occurring as I expected; I faced the unknown with a great deal of trepidation. I often felt lost when life events veered off course from my long-held expectations. But when I am able to hold these spiritual teachings close to my heart, I find I am less anxious about whatever current situation may be troubling me. I have, by no means, arrived at a state of equanimity that is completely independent of external factors, but I continue to work on shedding my overwhelming tendency to worry about things over which I have no control. It is a goal I try to keep in the forefront of my conscious mind.

It may be a common misinterpretation to think that letting go of expectations means becoming emotionally detached from people or events in our lives. In reality, by relinquishing our expectations of people or events, we are free to truly experience those relationships or events. If I am open to whatever happens in the present without being swayed by my attachment to the outcome, I have the opportunity to fully experience what happens, unburdened by preconceptions and their resulting disappointments.

Choosing your approach may involve changing your expectations. According to Buddhist belief, suffering is inevitable, but its sources can be identified and resolved. The Four Noble Truths of Buddhism posit that life involves suffering; the suffering is a product of three root delusions (attachments, anger, and ignorance); suffering can end by resolving our root delusions; and the Eight-Fold Noble Path of Buddhism prescribes the way to control our body and mind so that we help others instead of doing them harm and generate wisdom in our own mind, both of which lead to resolution of our suffering.[37] If our attachments and expectations are the source of our pain, then letting go of our attachments and expectations will relieve our pain.

For example, we can perpetuate our unhappiness by clinging to expectations about our loved one's health, such as "She's in her prime, so she shouldn't be sick." This kind of thought may generate anger, disappointment, sorrow, or other negative feelings that get in the way of being peacefully present with the person we love. If we release the expectation that people in their prime shouldn't get sick, then that particular aspect of our distress dissolves. If we are no longer fighting that expectation and its attendant negative emotions, we may become more able to respond helpfully to our loved one. No longer burdened by anger, sorrow, or disappointment, we will have more emotional capacity to feel close and connected to the person we love.

---

37 Peter Della Santina, *The Tree of Enlightenment: An Introduction to the Major Traditions of Buddhism* (Morristown, NJ: Yin-Shun Foundation, 1999).

Integrating Inconsistencies

I will not take "but" for an answer.
—Langston Hughes

For those of us who thrive on clarity and resolve, the clear-cut lines we have relied on in the past may seem to dissolve. Our world feels nebulous and contradictory. Somehow we need to find a way to become comfortable with that ambiguity.

When I was in law school, I thought it curious that a party in a case could offer alternative pleas, even if they were mutually exclusive. Disjunctive theories could proceed simultaneously. ("It couldn't have been me, because I was out of town. In the alternative, I was there, but it was self-defense.") It feels illogical to take two inconsistent positions at the same time. But sometimes we have to present two ideas as potentially true, not as exclusive of each other. I watched our rabbi do this artfully as he talked to Bill about "this and" that instead of "this but."

For example, consider these two approaches:

- "We are still hoping that your disease will stabilize, *but* if it doesn't, you need to talk to your wife about your wishes."
- "We are still hoping that your disease will stabilize, *and* at the same time, why don't you talk to your wife about your wishes, just in case?"

This may seem like an overly subtle distinction, but in the second example, one idea doesn't negate the other, the way it does in the first example. And for us, psychologically, this made a big difference. Somehow it didn't feel like a betrayal of hope to have these types of discussions. Even healthy people talk about arrangements "just in case."

Or consider a woman I knew who maintained her optimism about her chances for recovery even in the latest stages of her illness. She continued to assure her young daughter that "Mommy will be better soon."

She needed to believe this in order to sustain herself and to reassure her child. When it became clear that she was dying, her husband knew he needed to intervene to prevent his daughter from being blindsided. He had to weigh his wife's need for hope with his child's need for some preparation.

He told his daughter privately, "Mommy wants to believe so much that she will get better. She is not lying to you; she is wishing it with all of her heart. You need to know that she is very probably not going to get better, even though she wants to more than anything."

His daughter understood and did not appear surprised. He then told his wife about the conversation and asked her to make a similar acknowledgment while still holding on to her hope. He wanted his wife to say a few things to her daughter just in case, instead of only perpetuating unconvincing assurances.

She responded, talking with her daughter in a tender moment and saying, "I'm still hoping for a miracle, and just in case it doesn't happen, I want you to know how much I love you and how proud I am of you." She was then able to talk to her daughter about her hopes and dreams without specifically addressing the gravity of the situation.

Faith and Spirituality

> *Faith consists in believing when it is beyond the power of reason to believe.*
> —Voltaire

A quick stroll around any bookstore will reveal volumes of material about the role of faith and spirituality in confronting illness and other adversities. Whatever your belief system, you are likely to find a specific book that will speak to you on this subject. Individual approaches can be completely different, even among people who all consider themselves to be religious or spiritual.

Some people find comfort in the idea that a divine power will ultimately determine the outcome. ("God has a plan." "It is in God's hands.") Others have a more abstract concept of a presence in the universe that may influence events through positive energy or the power of community. Still others reject all of these concepts, believing in no higher power whatsoever. Not only are there many varied faiths, but there are also countless approaches within each of these faiths and denominations.

In times of crisis, people may be drawn closer to or turn away from religious or spiritual beliefs and practices in a way that differs from their previous tendencies. I know a couple who moved in separate directions when their son was killed in a car accident. The wife became more devout than ever, regularly attending her church for prayer and community. Meanwhile, her husband, bereft in anger and sorrow, found no comfort or meaning in his religion, which he felt had let him down. Neither approach was right; neither was wrong. Although each was respectful of the other's approach, the dissonance in their outlooks caused tension during a time that was already full of sadness and stress.

Sometimes we have our own inner conflicts about faith. If we reject it, we may feel guilty. If we devote all our emotional energy to the prospect of divine intervention, we may experience even greater disappointment or devastation if we feel our prayers have been to no avail. Whether we feel spiritually gratified may depend on what exactly has been the focus of our prayers or positive energy.

For example, we may petition for a specific outcome. ("Please don't let it be cancer." "Please make her better.") Or it may be a quality we hope for in ourselves. ("Please help me find strength." "Please let me handle this well.") Some people's prayers are not petitionary at all. ("Thank you for helping me cope with this situation." "Thank you for all the blessings I still have.") The feeling of having one's prayers "answered" may vary according to the specific intention or content of those prayers.

Some people feel no connection with religion but still have a cosmic awareness of something larger than themselves. It might be experienced as the force for good in the universe or as the positive energy of love and community. One of the most important things for people spiritually is to be at peace. People long for healing of body and healing of spirit or soul. Even those who have no particular religious practice or spiritual inclination look for meaning in our existence and in the way we experience our world.

Faith means believing in or trusting, usually in reference to a person, God, or religion. There are a variety of experiences of faith. Some people's faith takes a very literal form, guided by the teachings of their religion. They may feel comforted by reading the biblical story of Job, whose faith in God was not shaken— even by extreme hardship. Prayer may help them feel closer to God, and attending church, synagogue, or mosque may provide inspiration and comfort. Participating in a prayer circle may help them feel connected to and supported by people who share their faith.

Other people have a more abstract view of faith. For some, walking in the woods or on the beach may be a way to connect to God or a sense of the infinite power of the universe. For others, quiet reflection or reading poetry may help them tap into a deeper sense of connection or faith in the meaningfulness of the journey of life. Some people have their most powerful experiences of faith when people in their lives treat them with kindness and fidelity, restoring their faith in the goodness of the human spirit.

While there are myriad ways to experience faith, they all share the capacity to make a person feel supported, inspired, and part of a greater whole. There is not a right way to experience faith or God. Whatever form of faith comforts you is right for you.

One of the most challenging patients of my career so far was a man battling pancreatic cancer who was terrified of death. He did not believe in God, heaven, an afterlife, reincarnation, or any of the other abstract concepts that generally are consoling to people when they face the unknown. Nor did he believe that his presence on Earth would leave any lasting impression; he thought his life and work were ephemeral and meaningless. Lacking faith, he felt he was going alone into a void, his being obliterated. This was an extreme existential crisis, causing severe panic. Therapy or medications may be necessary to help alleviate a patient's emotional pain in such circumstances.

Internalizing Philosophies

*Once we see the world differently, we
seem to inhabit a new world.*
—ARNOLD GOLDBERG

As I work through my distress, I move to a place where the inspirational words I have been told and repeated become real for me.

It was not enough for me to say the right things. The true test was internalizing them into my being so that they were not just pithy aphorisms repeated merely to reassure me and others in my life. If you choose to integrate some of the concepts explored in this book, remember that they take practice, especially those that feel unnatural or unfamiliar. No one can pick up a guitar for the first time and expect to play it. There are chords to learn and awkward finger positions to master. For me, the goals of living in the present and reducing my worrying do not come easily and require a constant, continuing effort.

We are all able to recite the sound bites "Don't cross that bridge" and "Find the blessings." But they don't mean anything unless they travel from brain to heart and soul, where we hope they lodge and become part of our being.

Challenging the way you have always believed or acted may open up opportunities to think and experience things differently. If you always cross a green pasture in the same place, you will find yourself on a deep, entrenched path that may feel rutted and worn. Even if it has the benefit of familiarity, it may not be the most effective or positive way to go. By embarking on new paths, you may find more gratifying and helpful routes for your journey. When you find one that is satisfying, you might want to keep walking on this one for a while to get it established so that it becomes a part of you.

> Successful psychotherapy involves the internalization of healthy concepts about the self. It often starts with an idea or a cognitive concept, something that may sound good but feel foreign, such as "I am a person worthy of respect." Over time, the idea is internalized, essentially incorporated into the sense of self, so that it is no longer a thought but a deeper knowing. Occasionally this happens quickly, the result of an epiphany. More often it involves a subtle, evolving process of internal change that happens as a result of the relationship between patient and therapist.

> One need not be in therapy to internalize a philosophy. Acting as if the feeling or belief were true actually changes your neural networks and may gradually lead to its being true. One of my patients had very low self-esteem, which led her to accept disrespectful behavior from her employer and from her partner. After this problem was identified, she created a catchphrase to help remind herself of the new attitude she wanted to embrace: "I am a gem."

> She started to say this to herself whenever she became aware that she was feeling bad about the way someone was treating her. It helped her to change the way she responded to mistreatment, which in turn led to changes in the ways other people treated her. At first, she felt a little silly repeating, "I am a gem," but in time, she came to truly believe it, and her life has evolved to confirm to herself and others her tremendous value as a person.

Finding Joy

*For happiness one needs security, but joy can spring
like a flower even from the cliffs of despair.*
—Anne Morrow Lindbergh

One morning, as I was making coffee right before sitting down to work on this book, I was listening to a radio interview. The woman being interviewed had a son with severe disabilities. She described in detail the extensive care her child required and the way that she, on her own, had taken care of him and his five siblings. There came a point, she said, when she just could not do it anymore. She was completely overwhelmed and exhausted by the physical and emotional demands of her life. She thought she would break down if she had to do it one more day.

"And then," she declared, "I chose joy."

At that point, she changed her whole perspective on her life's circumstances. She willed herself to find the blessings and rewards in taking care of her son. She appreciated her son's abilities instead of focusing on his disabilities. She discovered the ways she could learn from her situation and grow as a person. She chose joy.

To me, this mother's experience was more than simple mind over matter or making lemons into lemonade. It was not about being in denial; rather, she scoped out the situation and made a conscious decision about living her life.

> This concept of "joy" is similar to the feeling I call "peace." For me, the highest state of contentment involves stillness. It doesn't mean I'm sitting still; I could be on a hike or dancing at a wedding or laughing with my friends. It doesn't need to involve special events; I could be writing on my computer while my family is working on their own projects in the next room, or I could be raking leaves in the autumn sunshine or listening to a patient in my office.

When I feel most content, I am fully present in whatever I'm doing, and I'm not struggling against myself. It's as if all the elements of my being are lined up in the same direction; body, intellect, heart, and soul are all engaged in the same activity with a common purpose. This congruence creates a stillness within, and that inner peacefulness is the state I experience as joy. As Laura wrote, happiness need not be an ingredient of joy.

How does one find peace in the midst of stressful life circumstances? One relaxes into it. Just as a cramped muscle relaxes with the right amount of stretching and massage, a cramped psyche relaxes when the environment offers enough support for you to breathe deeply and just go with the flow. By "environment," I mean everything from your attitude to the presence of friends and the way you treat your body. If your psyche stays cramped with chronic stress, you will have more physical and emotional difficulty than if you can interrupt the stress response and move forward freely.

It has not been instinctive for me to think about joy as a choice. If I even considered the subject at all in the past, I'm sure I thought about it as something that happens to you when everything in your life is right. But is that ever the case? Isn't there always something wrong? Even when we weren't facing the challenges of our loved one's illness, weren't there problems, disappointments, or frustrations that often prevented us from choosing joy?

Over the course of many months, I scoured book after book, looking for perspectives that might inspire me. One of the most powerful passages I read was this one from Naomi Remen's *Kitchen Table Wisdom*:

I had thought joy to be rather synonymous with happiness, but it seems now to be far less vulnerable than happiness. Joy seems to be a part of an unconditional wish to live, not holding back because life may not meet our preferences and expectations. Joy seems to be a function of the willingness to accept the whole, and to show up to meet with whatever is there. It has a kind of invincibility that attachment to any particular outcome would deny us...The willingness to win or lose moves us out of an adversarial relationship to life and into a powerful kind of openness. From such a position, we can make a greater commitment to life. Not only pleasant life, or comfortable life, or our idea of life, but all of life. [38]

When the dust first settled after Bill's diagnosis, I wondered whether I would ever be happy again. The answer to that was yes, but I think I experienced joy sooner and more often than the elusive happiness.

Joy feels more overarching than, and not as precarious as, happiness. It is a state of mind and a state of heart. Viewing joy as a decision leaves room to consciously acknowledge that, while everything may not be great in your life, you are going to choose it anyway. When we select other things in our lives—jobs, mates, friends, schools—we consider the alternatives, and ideally after introspection and reflection, we choose what is meaningful to us; we choose the course we think will be best. Being in a state of limbo, we cannot wait for an event to occur to cause us to be happy or content. The circumstance we most desperately want (our loved one's cure/survival/remission) may never happen, and so despite that prospect, we nonetheless must discover a way to live life with joy. Not only is this possible, but it is our obligation, as caregivers of our loved ones and architects of our own lives.

---

38 Rachel Naomi Remen, *Kitchen Table Wisdom: Stories That Heal* (New York: Riverhead, 1996), 171–2.

About the Authors

Laura Michaels, MA, JD, earned her undergraduate degree from Oberlin College. She received her law degree from the University of Denver, and her MA in counseling from Regis University.

A professional counselor in private practice, Ms. Michaels spent twenty years as the executive director of the Colorado Psychiatric Society (CPS). She was a founding member of the Colorado Behavioral Health Partnership and served on local and national mental health committees through the American Psychiatric Association (APA).

Claire Zilber, MD, received her BA in psychology from Haverford College, her medical degree from Thomas Jefferson University, and her psychiatric training at the University of Colorado. She also graduated from the psychodynamic psychotherapy program at the Denver Institute for Psychoanalysis.

Dr. Zilber is in private practice. She is also a clinical assistant professor in the University of Colorado's psychiatry department. She writes a regular column for CPS and APA publications, and she is on the faculty of the Professional/Problem-Based Ethics program at the Center for Personalized Education for Physicians.